WINNING THE WAR AGAINST

SICKNESS AND SEX IN DREAM

DANGEROUS AND EFFECTIVE PRAYERS AGAINST

SICKNESS, SPIRIT HUSBANDS (SEX IN DREAMS)

AND AFFLICTIONS

PRINCE HUBERT TATANG

(PRINCE) TATANG DJIOFACK HUBERT RONIS

Contacts: **+237- 79 71 62 90;**

+237-94 07 51 32

princeofj@gmail.com

DEDICATION

This book is dedicated to God the Father, the Son and the Holy Spirit.

To my sweet mother Kengni Madeleine, who sacrificed her livelihood to give me the best in life, who tilled the ground under rain and sun for my education,

To all those who contributed in one way or the other to my coming to the faith,

I love you all,

To my father in the ministry and his darling wife Rev. and Mrs Daniel,

To my Prophet Bishop Doctor David O. Oyedepo,

Not forgetting my sweet heart Doris for love, care and support in prayers.

CONTENTS

Acknowledgments   i

ACKNOWLEDGMENTS

TO JESUS THE MEDIATOR OF THE NEW COVENANT.
DEAR HOLY SPIRIT, THANK YOU, I ACKNOWLEDGE
YOUR GRACE, WISDOM, INSIGHTS, STRENGTH, LOVE
AND INSPIRATION FOR THE WRITING AND
PUBLISHING OF THIS BOOK.

JESUS YOU ARE MY ALL. TO YOU ALONE BE ALL THE
GLORY FOR ALL AGES. AMEN!

THANK YOU MY HEAVENLY FATHER FOR THIS
PRIVILEGE.

Thanks to all my pastors in China, Nigeria and in Cameroon,
And my sons in the Lord, Claude and his sweet heart Gisele for
their love and support in prayers,

To my wonderful mother Kengni Madeleine,

To the Man of God Rev. Doctor Tamo Achu,

Thanks to Pastor Arrey Ettah for reading through this book.

I am grateful to all those who have been a blessing to
me in one way or the other. I love you all.

INTRODUCTION

For I will restore health unto thee, and I will heal thee of thy wounds, saith the LORD, Jeremiah 30: 17
Beloved, I wish above all things that thou mayest prosper and be in health, even as thy soul prospereth,
3 John 2

Many are going through all manner of sufferings and afflictions around the world in these our days. No doubt, all the sufferings, wickedness and hatred we are facing in our time are already indicators of the end of this age, and consequently the heralding of the return of Christ. Yes, the world is drawing closer to the end, and no one except God and His Christ can –if they choose to- stop the chaos and turbulence all the world over, but there is a way of escape.

Whatever is going on cannot make the word of God void. As Christ Jesus our Lord and Master of the universe said, heaven (the sky) and earth can pass away, and will surely pass away, but not one jot of His written word will be broken or made of no effect.

Sicknesses, diseases and all kinds of new ailments visit our world year by year, and inflict the inhabitants of the earth. Yet the word of God stands true and sure: **"For I will restore health unto thee, and I will heal thee of thy wounds, saith the LORD"**.

1

Many are sick and afflicted around the globe, many have died of these terrible and incurable diseases and many go on living on drugs, yet the living and sure word of the unfailing God says (not suggest): **"Beloved, I wish above all things that thou mayest prosper and be in health, even as thy soul prospereth".**

Many sicknesses and diseases are said to be incurable and terminal, many of which have defied medical science and genius, yet the Holy Bible says; **"Bless Jehovah, O my soul; and all that is within me, *bless* His holy name. Bless Jehovah, O my soul, and forget not all His benefits; who forgives all your iniquities; who HEALS ALL your diseases"**(Psalms 103: 1-3).

So God heals all kinds of sicknesses that can attack and harass our mortal bodies as the Holy Spirit quickens us by the resurrection power of the Lord. We can be healed anywhere at any time, of any kind of disease. God has already made provision for our healing and healthy living in Christ by making Him die on the cross with our sins and sicknesses;

"Surely our diseases He did bear, and our pains He carried; whereas we did esteem Him stricken, smitten of God, and afflicted. But He was wounded because of our transgressions, He was crushed because of our iniquities: the chastisement of our welfare was upon Him, and with His stripes we were healed. All we like sheep did go astray, we turned everyone to his own way; and the LORD hath made to light on Him the iniquity of us all" Isa 53: 4-6 (JPS).

In actual facts, Christians, worshippers of the Living God, regenerated in God's image are not supposed to be sick, but if it happens, God requires us to pray in the Name of His Son Jesus Christ and He will heal us whatever the name of the ailment claimint our body, which is His own temple where He dwells.

> **<u>If</u> you <u>worship</u> me, the LORD your God, I will bless you with food and water and <u>take away all</u> your <u>sicknesses</u>,** Exodus 23: 25(GNB).
>
> **Are any among you in trouble? They should pray... Are any among you sick? They should send for the church elders, who will pray for them and rub olive oil on them in the name of the Lord. This prayer made in faith will heal the sick; the Lord will restore them to health, and the sins they have committed will be forgiven,** James 5: 13-14 (GNB). **Is any among you suffering? Let him pray... Is any among you sick? Let him call for the elders of the church; and let them pray over him, anointing him with oil in the name of the Lord: and the prayer of faith shall save him that is sick, and the Lord shall raise him up; and if he have committed sins, it shall be forgiven him,** James 5: 13-14 (ASV) .

PART ONE

UNDERSTANDING HEALING

Acts 20: 32 **And now, brethren, I commend you to God, and to the word of his grace, which is able to build you up, and to give you an inheritance among all them which are sanctified.**

Colossians 1: 12 **Giving thanks unto the Father, which hath made us meet to be partakers of the inheritance of the saints in light**

Matthew 15: 25-26 **Then came she and worshipped him, saying, Lord, help me. But he answered and said, It is not meet to take the children's bread, and to cast it to dogs**

Proverbs 15: 29 **The LORD is far from the wicked: but he heareth the prayer of the righteous.**

Proverbs 28: 9 **He that turneth away his ear from hearing the law, even his prayer shall be abomination.**

CHAPTER ONE

THE TRUTH

Jesus answered them, "You are mistaken because you don't know the Scriptures or God's power, Mat 22: 29

The truth is that God heals all kinds of sicknesses. The truth is that God can heal you. It is His will that you be healed, and live on without sickness. So, with God you can overcome sicknesses and all afflictions of satan including sex in dream, eating in dream and so on. As, the scripture says, if the Lord be for us, who (including satan and sicknesses) can be against us?

Many are suffering just because they don't know God. Some are in the church, but they are completely ignorant of the scriptures. Many are just following blind religion and blind leaders who have nothing of the living word to offer them. By the Holy Spirit, the apostle said, **"And now, brethren, I commend you to God, and to THE WORD of his grace, which is able to build you up, and to give you an inheritance among all them which are sanctified"**. He understood the place and virtue of the word of grace. There is no recovery without discovery. What you discover in scriptures determines what you recover in life and destiny.

All things are possible with God, including healing,

provided we ask Him by faith. God will not give you sickness when you asked for healing or for health. If your corrupted mentality makes you think that it is normal for you to be sick and afflicted though in the church, you will be. If you think it is normal for you or your child to live on drugs, that is exactly what you will get. What you know and what you believe is what shape your prayer life. You cannot ask your father for one million dollars unless you know he has and believe he will want to give you. God is reach, wealthy, All sufficient, All powerful and Unlimited, but we limit by our knowledge of Him. For we only ask to the limit of what we know He can do.

Many instead of asking God for their total healing and victory over sicknesses religiously ask God to help them bear their afflictions, because according to them, they must suffer in the flesh as Job. No men, Christ had not died at the time of Job; the price had not yet been paid. We are in the New Testament; renew your mind, lest satan rub you of your glorious Christianity on earth.

During our Radio program one day, a sister called in and asked us to pray for her to have enough grace to bear the demons and evil spirits tormenting her life. All the men of God in the studio broke into laughter. My colleague rightly told her, that though she needs grace to stands, she shouldn't be praying for the grace to bear them, but for the power to subdue and overcome them. We prayed for her, but I came to understand later, that that is where many of our problems lie. We think the wrong things (because of inadequate information), and we ask the wrong thing.

God gives you what you ask for. He will not give you fish when you ask for a stone, and vice versa. Hannah asked for a male child and got a male child. Daniel asked for revelation and received revelation. Elijah asked for fire, and fire came down from the Lord out of Heaven.

If you ask for the grace to carry your sickness the rest of your life, you will be given just that. If you ask for enough finances to keep paying your bills, He will do just that. As a Christian, your finances and resources are meant for good living and for His Kingdom promotion. God blesses you so you can contribute to the expansion of His Kingdom on earth, but because many of us have lost touch with our purpose on earth, satan devours it. For more understanding, read our book "DIVINE HEALING IS STILL POSSIBLE..."

ASK THE FATHER WHAT YOU WANT

"Ask, and you will receive; seek, and you will find; knock, and the door will be opened to you. For everyone who asks will receive, and anyone who seeks will find, and the door will be opened to those who knock. Would any of you who are fathers give your son a stone when he asks for bread? Or would you give him a snake when he asks for a fish? As bad as you are, you know how to give good things to your children. How much more, then, will your Father in heaven give good things to those who ask him! Matthew 7: 7-11 (GNB).

And in that day ye shall ask me nothing. Verily, verily, I say unto you, Whatsoever ye shall ask the Father in my name, he will give *it* you, John 16: 23

"When that day comes, you will not ask me for anything. I am telling you the truth: the Father will give you whatever you ask of him in my name. Until now you have not asked for anything in my name; ask and you will receive, so that your happiness may be complete, John 16: 23-24 (GNB).

God is a good Father who gives good things but to those who ask of Him believing that it will be as we so desire and have asked.

And you notice from all the above Biblical references that

God makes no difference as to the kind or nature or name of the sickness. Sickness is sickness and healing is healing. God gives us healing and sound health as we ask Him for it in prayers by the Name of Jesus Christ. You have to believe that He hears you, and ask Him to heal you of whatever sickness. You have to believe you can ride over sicknesses and live a sickness-free life, and ask Him to keep you healthy. Discover what the scriptures say about healing and health, and claim them for yourself and your loved ones.

No other religion will save you or help you out. You will do yourself a favor by believing in Jesus and become a child a God; that is, a Christian. Many foolish religions and sects have deceived many that God has no son. Well dear, Jesus Christ is well alive; and is the Son of the Living God; the sole Creator of the whole universe. The One to whom we will all give account of what we did here on earth. So as you seek to live healthy and happy on earth, seek and thrive above all odds to spend eternity in peace and joy with the Living and Loving God in Heaven. Without Jesus no one will get there.

The world leaders and kings are in a great mistake, joining evil and pernicious cults to be in power for a few days or decades, turning down God's offer for salvation, trading down the sacrifice of the Son of God for their escape. It will be terrible on the judgment day. In fact, I am sure many of them are having their share in hell already. I shared in my book **"WHY MUST I**

BECOME A CHRISTIAN?", as the Lord took me to hell on the 17th of April 2013 at 2 am. It was terrible and pathetic, as I saw souls of men wailing and crying for help, but it was impossible to help them out. Get that book and learn the truth about Christianity.

So the prayer of faith is one of the mediums to get healed and ride over sicknesses and diseases the rest of our lives.

REVELATION

However, Prayer is not enough to secure the healing and health we need. Of course, divine healing and divine health are both God's provisions for His children on the earth made available and possible by the death of His Son Jesus Christ on the cross more than two thousand years ago. Yet lack of understanding has robbed and continues to rob many in the church of these wonderful gifts and blessings of God.

Revelation is the proper understanding of the written scriptures. It is having insight into what God says and appropriating it rightly for our profiting. They will be no revelation of the word of God until we go for the word; reading and searching the scriptures.

Revelation comes as we read, study, meditate and reason with the word of God. Not reasoning the word (questioning its integrity, doubting, trying to understand God with your mind and intelligence), but reasoning with it (digging it out, questioning what it means, asking questions) knowing that it is spirit and speaks.

Many continue to see healing as a promise that will be fulfilled someday, maybe when Christ comes. As for divine health, it is absolutely impossible to many. In some parts of the world, you are seen as a blasphemer when you talk of healing and sound health without medication or medical intervention due to ignorance. For my people, says the Lord, are destroyed for lack of knowledge (Hosea 4: 6). For some years now I have vowed, from the day I cut the revelation of divine healing and sound health in Christ, never to lie on a hospital bed. I have come to a point that sickness is totally a stranger to me now. I feel strange and hurt when I see a child of God sick and going through the same pains with unbelievers, the worst is when the accept it and take it normal. Why then did Christ die on the cross? Did He die in vain? Many accept that Christ dealt with our sins on the cross, but how about our sicknesses? If sickness came into the world through sin, then it should go when sin is rooted out of our lives. Do the scriptures not mean what they say? In the Old Testament, God promised us healing and a life of blessing, fruitfulness, and freedom from all the sicknesses that are in the world. The promised was fulfilled in Christ Jesus:

Thou shalt be blessed above all people: there shall not be male or female barren among you, or among your cattle.

And the LORD will take away from thee all sickness, and will put none of the evil diseases of Egypt, which thou knowest, upon thee... Deuteronomy 7: 14-15.

When Jesus came, He healed a lot of sicknesses. People were still suffering of afflictions because the problem of sin had not been solved. Sickness was permitted to touch the Old Testament Jews because the savior had not come, because of their rebellion and disobedience to the law, they were under the curse of the law, which is actually the root-cause of sickness. You can get that from Deuteronomy 28

NOTE: As you read through, you may think God gives sickness. Actually God permits the avenger to touch you when through disobedience you get out of His protective umbrella.

Sickness came into the world through sin and disobedience, but it was taken care of by God through the cross. Jesus took away the curse from earth so that those who believe in Him are spared of its works;

John 3: 16: **For God so loved the world, that he gave his only begotten Son, that whosoever believeth in him should not perish, but have everlasting life.**

Isaiah 53: 5: **But he was wounded for our transgressions, he was bruised for our iniquities: the chastisement of our peace was upon him; and with his stripes we are healed.**

Isaiah 33: 24: **And the inhabitant shall not say, I am sick: the people that dwell therein shall be forgiven their iniquity.**

Galatians 3: 9-10, 13: **So then they which be of faith are blessed with faithful Abraham. For as many as are of the works of the law are under the curse: for it is written, Cursed is every one that continueth not in all things which are written in the book of the law to do them... Christ hath redeemed us from the curse of the law, being made a curse for us: for it is written, Cursed is every one that hangeth on a tree.**

CHAPTER TWO

THE STARTING POINT

YOU MUST BE SAVED

Are you saved? Salvation is the starting point for divine healing and every of God's blessings. It is new birth that frees you and sets you on high above satan and his assaults.

Jesus cannot do anything for you until you believe in Him and get saved. Because healing, health, wealth, a bright career, long life and whatever you may boast of is a waste without Christ. Having all the world put together without being saved is madness and folly, because at the end, you will land in hell for all eternity. God wants you in Heaven at all cost. It is far better to end in Heaven blind, footless, handless or homeless than to own all the duplexes of the world, have two eyes and land in hell. Of course Jesus still heals the blind and turns the wretched and poor into wealthy people, but the salvation of your soul is God's heartbeat. While many are blaming and cursing God for having allowed sickness into the world, God is angry with them for having rejected and despised His Son Jesus Christ, and thereby tread down so great a salvation. Sometimes, as I witness to people about the love, goodness and omnipotence of Jehovah, many ask why God could not take away sickness, and sin completely and even kill satan if He were so loving and All-powerful as we preach. You don't need to ask why, simply accept the way of escape God has provided for you.

Jesus answered, Verily, verily, I say unto thee, Except a man be born again, he cannot see the kingdom of God, John 3: 3.

If thou shalt confess with thy mouth the Lord Jesus, and shalt believe in thine heart that God hath raised him from the dead, thou shalt be saved. Because with the heart man believeth unto righteousness, and with the mouth confession is made unto salvation, Romans 10: 9-10.

If you do not receive Jesus the only Savior of all mankind, you will not enter the kingdom of God, despite your good works. Salvation is by grace through faith (**Ephesians 2: 8-9**).

No tradition, no religion, no prophet or sacrifice can save you from sin and hell. Even if doctors cure you, you can only get true healing and health from God. Besides, they cannot offer you the forgiveness of your sins that only Jesus freely offers. Your sect and religion cannot save you, your bank account and your cars and houses will remain on earth. How about you? Where will your soul be? Only Jesus Christ will save you from death, hell and judgment to come!

Come to Jesus now **"for there is ONE GOD, and ONE MEDIATOR between God and men, the man CHRIST JESUS. Who GAVE HIMSELF A RANSOM FOR ALL...Wherefore**

HE IS ABLE also to SAVE them to the uttermost that COME UNTO GOD BY HIM, seeing he ever liveth to make intercession for them "-1 Timothy 2: 5, Hebrews 7: 25.

Jesus freely offers you free forgiveness for all your sins and guarantees you eternity with God if you believe in Him and turn away from your ways, and accept Him as your Savior. Salvation is the base of healing. All God's blessings are rooted in salvation, including the healing, prosperity, marriage, children and promotion you are looking for.

PART TWO

UNDERSTANDING THE PRAYER OF HEALING

Matthew 7: 7-8: **Ask, and it shall be given you…**
For every one that asketh receiveth

John 14: 13-14: **And whatsoever ye shall ask in**
my name, that will I do, that the Father may be
glorified in the Son. If ye shall ask any thing in my
name, I will do it.

Isaiah 1: 15-17: **And when ye spread forth your**
hands, I will hide mine eyes from you: yea, when ye
make many prayers, I will not hear: your hands are
full of blood. Wash you, make you clean; put away the
evil of your doings from before mine eyes; cease to do
evil; Learn to do well

Isaiah 59: 1-2: **Behold, the LORD's hand is not**
shortened, that it cannot save; neither his ear heavy,
that it cannot hear: But your iniquities have
separated between you and your God, and your sins
have hid his face from you, that he will not hear.

BASIC PRINCIPLES AND REREQUISITES TO ANSWERED PRAYERS

Ephesians 6: 18: **Praying always with all prayer and supplication in the Spirit, and watching thereunto with all perseverance and supplication for all saints**

I- PRAYER IS INSPIRED AND DYNAMIC

Understand that prayer is a spiritual and dynamic art. Prayer is not a recitation; it is not a mere repetition. Thus, the prayers proposed in this book are inspired by the Holy Spirit to help you in specific circumstances. You're not obliged or forced to recite them all your life. You should not just recite them as a class one pupil. Declare them with all your being and all your energy; let it spring from your heart.

Moreover, God expects you to grow in your faith and in your prayer life. The more you grow in God's word and in your relationship and communion with the Holy Spirit, the more you will receive His help in prayer in order to formulate your own prayers. **"Likewise the Spirit also helps our infirmities, for we**

know not what we should pray as we ought: But the Spirit itself makes intercession for us with groaning which cannot be uttered, and he that searches the hearts knows what is the mind of the Spirit, because he makes intercession for the saints according to the will of God", Romans 8:26-27.

When God pours upon you His Spirit of grace and supplication that He has promised us, you are strengthened I your inner man and inspired in your prayers:

"And I will pour upon the house of David and on the inhabitants of Jerusalem a spirit of grace and supplication and they shall look upon me whom they have pierced ..." Zechariah 12:10.

So, prayer is from your heart. It is something born out of an earnest desire; something you want it at all cost. It is not trying it to see if it will work. If that is the case, expect no result. You must pray because God is your only source and you dearly and sincerely need what you are asking. However, you can advise or introduce this prayer book to someone who is sick or suffering an affliction. Use it as long as you can, only avoid photocopy or reproduction. The works of the Spirit of God should not be pirated or copied. Instead, contact us for any need and assistance; we're at your service 24/24h, and seven days on seven (7/7).

The prayers in this book are inspired, effective and endued with the power and anointing of the Holy Spirit of God if you believe. The power and anointing of the Holy Spirit will be released as you pray, and all satanic oppressions and yokes over your life will be broken in the Mighty Name of Jesus. So, do not just recite the prayers, do not just repeat them. Pray, confess and declare these prayers with conviction, faith and authority. Be angry against that disease or affliction harassing you. You can also do this for someone who is near or far from you mentioning his name and the name of his disease. If possible, ask the patient on the phone to receive Jesus as Lord and Savior before praying.

II- REPENTANCE IS INDISPENSABLE

He who conceals his sins shall not prosper, but whoever confesses and forsakes them shall obtain mercy, Proverbs 28: 13.

Come and hear, all you who fear God, and I will declare what he has done for my soul. I cried unto him with my mouth, And He was extolled with my tongue. IF I REGARD INIQUITY IN MY HEART, THE LORD WILL NOT hear me. But verily God has heard me, He has attended to the voice of my prayer. Blessed be God, who has not turned away my prayer, nor His mercy from me, Psalms 66: 16-20.

Secret and non-confessed sins can constitute a blockage to our prayers. That is why sincere and total repentance is the base in prayer. Do not hide pretend before God because He sees everything. Confess them to Him and sincerely repent. Repentance is the first step to being born again. Repentance means to make a U-turn. That is turning away from your sins and sinful habits, with a promise to God never to return to it. It therefore means you must be born again because every blessing of the Kingdom of God is a reserved of the redeemed, the sanctified in Christ. Healing and answers to prayers are for God's children. God does not answer the sinner because He is too pure to behold on iniquity, unless the sinner turns from his sins and forsakes them. Willful sin is a hindrance to prayers. **"Behold, the LORD's hand is not shortened, that it cannot save; neither his ear heavy, that it cannot hear: But your iniquities have separated between you and your God, and your sins have hid his face from you, that he will not hear"**, Isaiah 59: 1. But once you confess and turn from your sins, He will completely erase and forget them even if men continue to condemn you: **"I, even I, am he that blotteth out thy transgressions for mine own sake, and will not remember thy sins"**, Isaiah 43: 25.

David said**, "Bless the LORD, O my soul, and forget not all his benefits: Who forgiveth all thine iniquities; who healeth all thy diseases"** Psalms 103: 2-3.

So forgiveness of our sins precedes healings of our bodies. I am not saying you should be guilty. But if you know you are living in sin, if you know that you have turned away from the truth of God's word, don't pretend. Stop going from pastor to pastor, from prophet to prophet, from deliverance house to another, you can't bribe or manipulate God. He is the same GOD all those pastors and prophets are serving, unless they are prophets of Baal. Simply repent and turn back to God.

Besides, even if by the anointing and faith of the man of God you get healed in your sins and rebellion, and you continue in it, be ready for more trouble because that demon will return with seven spirits more wicked than himself and you will regret the rest of your life.

"Afterward Jesus findeth him in the temple, and said unto him, Behold, thou art made whole: sin no more, lest a worse thing come unto thee" John 5: 14.

Why did Jesus take time to ask him to repent genuinely and turn to sin no more; that is to change?

BECAUSE **"When the unclean spirit is gone out of a man, he walketh through dry places, seeking rest, and findeth none. Then he saith, I will return into my house from whence I came out; and when he is come, he findeth it empty, swept, and garnished. Then goeth he, and taketh with himself seven other spirits more wicked than himself, and they enter in and dwell there: and the last state of that man is worse than the first. Even so shall it be also unto this wicked generation"**. Mathieu 12: 43-45

You are not obliged to confess your sins to men; you may

do that if you are led because it is scriptural. However, the best way is to settle it with your Heavenly Father who alone forgives and blots out our sins. Right now, if you feel you have departed from the Lord, look for a quiet and calm place where you are alone and pray this prayer of repentance and reconciliation with God if you wish to:

[**My Lord and my God, I come to you by the blood of Your Son Jesus as I am, in the Name of Jesus. I acknowledge that I have sinned against you and against men. Receive me and forgive me all my sins that I have committed against you and against man. I repent sincerely for ...** (mention them to Him and sincerely confess and repent). **Lord Jesus, I admit, and believe you died for my sins. And that you rose again from the dead for my justification according to Romans chapter 4 verse 25, and in you I have redemption and forgiveness for all my sins by your blood according to Ephesians chapter 1 verse 7. I agree and confess that you are my only Lord and personal Savior. Make me a child of God and write my name in your book of life. I rededicate my life to you this day. Save my soul and deliver my life from the pit. Give me your Spirit today, fill and baptize me in the Holy Ghost and help me to follow you the rest of my days on earth. Thank you dear Lord, for forgiving me in Jesus' Precious Name. Thank you Holy Spirit because you now dwell in me and my life will never be the same again in the Mighty Name of Jesus. Now that I am forgiven and saved, help me Holy Spirit, give me the grace to** forgive and love all those who have offended me in the Name of our Lord Jesus Christ. Amen!]

Now, you are forgiven. Forget your past. Forgive yourself and forgive all those who ever hurt you in any way. But, return no longer to it, like the man Jesus delivered from 38 years of affliction by the pool: **"Afterward Jesus findeth him in the temple, and said unto him, Behold, thou art made whole: sin no more, lest a worse thing come unto thee"**, John 5: 14. Receive the grace to follow and serve God in the Mighty Name of Jesus Christ. Amen!

III- FAITH IS THE KEY

Jesus saith unto her, Said I not unto thee, that, if thou wouldest believe, thou shouldest see the glory of God? Jean 11. 40

NOW FAITH is the substance of things hoped for, the evidence of things not seen... But without faith it is impossible to please him: for he that cometh to God must believe that he is, and that he is a rewarder of them that diligently seek him, Hebrews 11: 1, 6.

As soon as Jesus heard the word that was spoken, he saith unto the ruler of the synagogue, Be not afraid, ONLY BELIEVE, Marc 5: 36.

Do not fret because of words and reports of men. Do not

fear death; do not fear sickness or anything. Do not even think about those who have died of the same thing that you are suffering. Your case is different if you believe. Do not fear what your doctors say and the results of your tests. It is not the disease that kills; rather it is ignorance and unbelief that kill most people. Yes, many have died of AIDS, yet many are alive with the same AIDS for years without any problem. It's not AIDS or cancer that killed them; it was their ignorance and unbelief. Many have been healed and continue to be healed of AIDS by the power of God through faith in Jesus Christ.

However, it is not prayer alone that heals; it is faith in Jesus and His Word. Jesus said (John 11: 4): **"This sickness is not unto death, but for the glory of God, that the Son of God might be glorified thereby."** Just believe that you will live and be healed. So when you pray, believe and accept you're healed by faith, and you will see it. If you expect to see it before believing, it is unbelief, and you will never see anything. Because **"FAITH is the substance of things hoped for... of things not seen." "Therefore I say unto you, What things soever ye desire, when ye pray, BELIEVE THAT YE RECEIVE them, and ye shall have them."** After the prayer, ignore the symptoms and pain, agree that God has heard and healed you, and continue reading, rereading and meditating on a verse of Scripture that addresses your situation, which confirms your healing as 1 Peter 2 : 24.

What is faith?

Faith is accepting God's word as true and real, regardless of your situation. Faith is agreeing with God concerning what you want. Faith is accepting that by His stripes I am already healed, whether you see a sign or not.

Faith is behaving God's word. It is acting on the word of God. The same way you accept the doctor's report without seeing what he says you are suffering of, that is how you should accept God's own report and behave as if you were never sick.

If you are suffering of spirit husband or sex in dreams, it is a satanic affliction. Just put in your mind that they can't touch you any longer because you are born of God. Most of our troubles and afflictions are as a result of unbelief and ignorance. Satan is not afraid of your prayer and fasting, but he dreads your knowledge of God and the revelation of who you really are in Christ. In Christ you are higher spirit than him and his demons, talk less of his agents the witches and wizards who sleep you in the nights. Now concerning the believers in Christ, it is written:

We know that whosoever is born of God sinneth not; but he that is begotten of God keepeth himself, and that wicked one TOUCHETH him NOT. (1 Jon 5: 18).

It was not Jesus' fasting that gave Him victory over satan during His temptation hour. Rather it was His revelation and mastery of **"It is written".** He never had to bind satan, He simply shot the sword of the Spirit at him, which satan cannot resist. Get armed with your sword, and you sure of your sweat less victory over that fool;

> **"And take the helmet of salvation, and the sword of the Spirit, which is the word of God"** Ephesians 6: 17.

Being born again is not enough to overcome satan. As you take the helmet of salvation which is your new birth, you now need the sword to conquer. Your new birth (helmet of salvation) is the defensive, which is not enough to win in any battle. You need now the offensive, the sword of the Spirit of God, with which you will fight and win the fight.

Beloved, we are in the era of knowledge. GO FOR KNOWLEDGE. Stop running after miracles and laying of hands. Sit down with your Bible and get equip. remember we are in the last days. What is to happen in the last days?

> **And it shall come to pass in the last days, that the mountain of the LORD's house shall be established in the top of the mountains, and shall be exalted above the hills; and all nations shall flow unto it. And many people shall go and say, Come ye, and let us go up to the mountain of the LORD, to the house of the God of Jacob; and HE WILL TEACH US OF HIS WAYS, and we will walk in his paths: for out of Zion shall go forth the LAW, and THE WORD of the LORD from Jerusalem.** Isaiah 2: 2-3

> **"They shall not hurt nor destroy in all my holy mountain: for the earth shall be full of the KNOWLEDGE of the**

27

LORD, as the waters cover the sea" Isaiah 11: 9.

And WISDOM and KNOWLEDGE shall be the stability of thy times, and strength of salvation: the fear of the LORD is his treasure. Isaiah 33: 6.

So, whatever be the affliction you are facing, pray the prayers in this book with understanding and authority, being conscious of what is written concerning you. Declare what is written, and henceforth, when anything happens to you, when you see or hear anything threatening, just confidently declare what is written.

IV-   THE NAME OF JESUS

Wherefore God also hath HIGHLY EXALTED Him, and given Him a name which is above every name: That AT THE NAME OF JESUS every knee should bow, of things in heaven, and things in earth, and things under the earth; And that every tongue should confess that Jesus Christ is Lord, to the glory of God the Father, Philippians 2: 9-11
And whatsoever ye shall ask IN MY NAME, that will I do, that the Father may be glorified in the Son... Ye have not chosen me, but I have chosen you, and ordained you, that ye should go and bring forth fruit, and that your fruit should remain: that whatsoever ye shall ask of the Father IN MY

NAME, he may give it you... And in that day ye shall ask me nothing. Verily, verily, I say unto you, WHATSOEVER ye shall ASK the Father IN MY NAME, he will give it you. Hitherto have ye asked nothing IN MY NAME: ASK, and ye shall receive, that your joy may be full, John 14: 13, 15: 16; 16: 23-24.

The name of Jesus is a sure guarantee for us in prayer. It is a surety for answers to our prayers. Sometimes, God give us some things, not because of ourselves, nor just because we ask, but because of the Name of His beloved Son that is invoked. Whenever that Name is invoked, God remembers His obedience and ultimate sacrifice on the cross for mankind. When the Name is invoked in prayer with faith and understanding, the forces of hell take flight while the angels of God show up and stand to our attention. You do not need to go through long ways to get answers to your prayers. It is not written anywhere in the Bible that we should come to God through any saint whatsoever. It is ignorance and pure religion. Jesus is the only way through which we are to come to the Father and obtain whatever we request. We ourselves are God's saints on earth. Sinners and the unsaved are to know God through us, and be reconciled the Father through us as legal representatives of Jesus Christ the King of kings and Lord of lords; that is, through our testimony and witnessing. We point them to the Father while we live, and once we depart our job is completely and irrevocably over. We are not plead the departed (the dead in the name of saints) to get a favor from our Heavenly Father, who loves us and gives "good things to those who ask Him".

He did not say He gives good things to those who ask His mother or disciples, it is foolishness and madness. That you are sick, instead of commanding that nonsense disease by the power in the Name of Jesus to leave your life, you are wasting your time and energy enchanting saints and angels to help you. Do you know how much it pains and grieves God's heart and His Spirit any time you do that? Anyway, I will not blame you, it is simply because you are not born again, neither are you filled with the Holy Spirit. You keep blindly following religion and men's doctrines. You pay more attention to men's and church doctrines and dogmas than to the word of God. And you know what? Satan is very happy because lack of Knowledge destroys (Hosea 4: 6). Listen to the pure word of God;

> **If ye then, being evil, know how to give good gifts unto your children, how much more shall YOUR FATHER which is IN HEAVEN GIVE GOOD THINGS to THEM that ASK HIM?** Matthew 7: 11

> **Ye have not chosen me, but I have chosen you, and ordained you, that ye should go and bring forth fruit, and that your fruit should remain: that whatsoever ye shall ask of the Father IN MY NAME, he may give it you... Hitherto have ye asked nothing IN MY NAME: ASK, and ye shall receive, that your joy may be full** (John 15: 16; 16: 24. Be free from

the bondage of religion in Jesus Name. May you be loosed now and your eyes be opened in Jesus Precious Name! Amen!

Only Jesus rose from the death and is alive forever at the right hand of the Father to intercede for us. He alone is qualified by His death on the cross to obtain for us God's favor and blessings. He Alone offers forgiveness for sins. It is by His own stripes that we are healed (Isaiah 53: 5; 1 Peter 2: 24).

All other prophets and saints are death and gone. And it's really crazy, and waste of precious time looking for a third mediator who will ask Jesus to ask the Father to give us what we need. What a long way! Don't you know you're free to come directly to God for everything you need? O my people perish for lack of knowledge!

Therefore being JUSTIFIED by faith, WE HAVE PEACE with God through OUR LORD JESUS CHRIST: By whom also we have ACCESS by faith into this grace wherein we stand, and rejoice in hope of the glory of God. ... LET US therefore COME BOLDLY unto the throne of grace, that we may OBTAIN mercy, and find grace to help in time of need... Having therefore, BRETHREN, boldness to enter into the holiest by THE BLOOD OF JESUS, By a new and living way, which he hath consecrated for US, through the veil, that is to say, his flesh; And having an HIGH PRIEST over the house of God; LET US DRAW NEAR with a true heart in full

assurance of faith, having our hearts sprinkled from an evil conscience, and our bodies washed with pure water, Romans 5: 1-2, Hebrews 4: 16, 10: 19-22 .

Beloved, have you heard? Do you really understand? Being justified here means being made righteous, being sanctified and made holy before God by the blood of the lamb. If you are born again, know that you were justified, made righteous and holy before God and His angels at new birth. What qualifies you for free access to God the Father through faith in His son Jesus Christ, and by His Spirit who dwells in you, which is given at new birth.

The scriptures do not say that you have access to God through Jesus' mother, His apostles and His grandmother, but that you and I **"HAVE PEACE with God through OUR LORD JESUS CHRIST: By whom also we have ACCESS by faith into this grace wherein we stand."** By whom do we have this access? By Jesus Christ, the Son of the Living God who gave Himself for us, for it is by Him that we have by faith access to the grace of God.

Now, God invites us in **Hebrews 4: 16** to draw near (individually, by ourselves) to the throne of grace, as He also invites us in **Isaiah 1: 18 "Come now, and let us reason together, saith the LORD."**

According to Hebrews 10: 19-22, we brothers and sisters in Christ, saints of God on earth, have **"boldness to enter into the** holiest by **THE BLOOD OF JESUS, By a new and living way, which he hath consecrated for US, through the veil, that is to say, his flesh"** and we also have a " **HIGH PRIEST over the house of God."** This priest is neither Mary nor all the departed saints joined together, it is He who died for us, the very One who said, **"Ye have not chosen me, but I have chosen you, and ordained you, that ye should go and bring forth fruit, and that your fruit should remain: that whatsoever ye shall ask of the Father IN MY NAME, he may give it you."**

We are children of God, and I do not see why my daughter or my son I love will pass through my mother or my servants to obtain school fess. Unless he (or she) is an unruly and rebellious child who wants to manipulate his way through the sympathy of others. But it is not so with God. He either approves you or you are rejected, and no one apart from Jesus can change His mind.

Beloved, stop coming to your God like a beggar or a criminal. He is ashamed and disappointed every time you look for mediators while the Name of His Son answers to everything. Jesus paid the full price for your sins of the past, of now and tomorrow. You are not given a license to go on sinning freely, but know that Jesus never ceases to intercede for you before the Father, that He may grant you what you ask, even what you do not deserve. Being guilty and miserable all the time you will never help you. Seeing yourself as a sinner all the time is not holiness. Holiness is living and walking in the fear of God, with confidence and the

33

consciousness that all your sins and transgressions have been totally cleansed, and you are a new creation; a new man in Christ.

In Christ, all your sins are taken care of: **My little children, these things write I unto you, that ye sin not. And if any man sin, we have an advocate with the Father, Jesus Christ the righteous: And he is the propitiation for our sins: and not for ours only, but also for the sins of the whole world. And hereby we do know that we know him, if we keep his commandments,** 1 John 2: 1-3.

There are no two ways to God our Loving Creator, **"For there is ONE GOD, and ONE MEDIATOR between God and men, the man CHRIST JESUS; Who gave himself a ransom for ALL... But this man, because he continueth ever, hath an unchangeable priesthood. Wherefore HE IS ABLE also to save THEM to the uttermost THAT COME UNTO GOD BY HIM, seeing he ever liveth to make intercession FOR THEM"**, 1 Timothy 2: 5, Hebrews 7: 24-25.

I know that many are already so indoctrinated and closed up that they will not accept the truth even when God Himself speaks to them, they refuse to change and embrace the truth. I write not to judge or criticize, I write not against any movement or people, but by the Spirit of our God, your God and my God, your Heavenly Father and mine, I wrote to help you enjoy better your Christian walk on earth and enjoy better results and answers to your prayers.

In Hosea 4: 6, God laments, **"My people are destroyed for lack of knowledge: because thou hast rejected knowledge, I will also reject thee, that thou shalt be no priest to me: seeing thou hast forgotten the law of thy God, I will also forget thy children."**

So, for the sake of your children and your children's children, accept this truth and change the way you pray, and the way you relate to God. We are talking about effective prayers and not doctrines or denominations. It is not a particular church you attend or belong to, but what you must do to get your prayers answered and speedily. So if you desire a change in your prayer life and in your Christian life in general, change your approach to God and your attitude in prayer, and God will change His attitude and His approach towards you, and your prayers will bring you better results.

In conclusion, **"For there is ONE GOD, and ONE MEDIATOR between God and men, the man CHRIST JESUS...Wherefore HE IS ABLE also to save THEM to the uttermost THAT COME UNTO GOD BY HIM, seeing he ever liveth to make intercession FOR THEM".**

"Verily, verily, I say unto you, WHATSOEVER ye shall ASK the Father IN MY NAME, he will give it you. Hitherto have ye asked nothing IN MY NAME: ASK, and ye shall

receive, that your joy may be full ".

V-   THE WORD OF GOD IS THE SOURCE AND SEED OF YOUR HEALING

"Jesus saith unto him, Go thy way; thy son liveth. And the man believed THE WORD that Jesus had spoken unto him, and he went his way", John 4: 50.

My son, attend to MY WORDS; incline thine ear unto MY SAYINGS. Let them not depart from thine eyes; keep them in the midst of thine heart. For they are life unto those that find them, and health to all their flesh. Proverbs 4: 20-22.

When the even was come, they brought unto him many that were possessed with devils: and he cast out the spirits with HIS WORD, and healed all that were sick, Mathieu 8: 16.

As we have already said, the word of God is the source and the seed of every miracle and every transformation that any human needs in his life on the earth. We know that God created everything by His word and He sustains the universe by the word of His power, including my life and yours **(Hebrews 1: 3; 11: 3)**.

Without His word, your marriage has no support, your family has no stand, your health has no ground nor hope. Listen to this: **"Through faith we understand that the worlds were framed by the word of God... and upholding all things by the word of his power"** (Hebrews 11: 3, Hebrews 1: 3). God Himself has this to say about His words: "**For as the rain cometh down, and the snow from heaven, and returneth not thither, but watereth the earth, and maketh it bring forth and bud, that it may give seed to the sower, and bread to the eater: SO SHALL MY WORD be that GOETH FORTH OUT OF MY MOUTH: it shall not return unto me void, but IT SHALL ACCOMPLISH that which I please, and IT SHALL PROSPER in the thing whereto I SENT IT"** (Isaiah 55: 10-11).

The word of God that you read and believe acts in your life and accomplish His will and His good intentions (plans) in your life, your health, your future, your marriage, your children, your finances, your education, and everything that concerns you. So, to effectively pray for healing or any other thing, locate a Bible passage that contains promise of God for you, confirming what you need. That is why all the prayers in this book always start with relevant Biblical passages. If you're new in Christ, if you do not know the Biblical passages dealing with the problem you are facing in your life, take a scripture like **John chapter 3 verse 16**, which dealing with salvation and eternal life, answers to all of man's needs, or also **Jeremiah 29** verse **11**, which also covers all aspects of our lives.

" For God so loved the world that he gave his only begotten Son, that whosoever believeth in him should not perish, but have everlasting life" John 3: 16.

" For I know the plans I have for you, says the Lord, thoughts

of peace and not of evil, to give you a future and a hope"
Jeremiah 29: 11.

VI-   THERE IS NO DISTANCE IN THE SPIRIT

It is also very important to understand and know that there is no distance or limit the spirit realm. Prayers know no bounds. The same prayers that you pray for yourself and God answers, you can also do the same for someone in India, America and Japan and God still visits the person instantly right where he is. Remember this nobleman who came to invite Jesus to come and pray for his son. Jesus did not need to go there, He just sent His word and the problem was solved on instantly as this man believed **(John 4: 46-54):**

So Jesus came again into Cana of Galilee, where he made the water wine. And there was a certain nobleman, whose son was sick at Capernaum. When he heard that Jesus was come out of Judaea into Galilee, he went unto him, and besought him that he would come down, and heal his son: for he was at the point of death.

Then said Jesus unto him, Except ye see signs and wonders, ye will not believe. The nobleman saith unto him, Sir, come down ere my child die. Jesus saith unto him, Go thy way; thy son liveth. And the man believed the word that Jesus had spoken unto him, and he went his way. And as he was

now going down, his servants met him, and told him, saying, Thy son liveth. Then enquired he of them the hour when he began to amend. And they said unto him, Yesterday at the seventh hour the fever left him. So the father knew that it was at the same hour, in the which Jesus said unto him, Thy son liveth: and himself believed, and his whole house. This is again the second miracle that Jesus did, when he was come out of Judaea into Galilee.

The word will work for you, and the power of God will avail for you and your loved ones no matter your location and distance. Just believe and you will see the Glory of God in your life and family.

Many times, as soon as the doctor gives a diagnosis, the children of God do not ask what the Great Physician, Doctor of all doctors, Doctor of all nurses, the Supreme Chief of all surgeons has to say in His report: **His word**. The medical report is not and must not always be final. Doctors are doing a great and good job the world over, I love them and do appreciate them, however their reports are simply the analysis of the situation, and the word of God that controls the universe gives us the solution, and guaranties alone our total deliverance. Moreover, the doctor treats, and it is God who truly heals and offers sound and lasting health.

No matter your location, God's power can still locate you and heal you. That is why you can get your healing via telephone call, Radio or TV teachings and prayers. The power of God is instant, swift and unlimited. No immigration officer or expert can stop it. Many people have obtained their deliverance and healing as we pray on Radio or Television. Others have received their miraculous touch through books, tapes and video messages of anointed Men and Women of God. You can still contact the healing power of the Holy Spirit as you read this book. All it takes is faith.

It therefore means that you can still call us right now for prayers; as we pray for you on phone, you will be instantly healed and delivered. Our contacts are found at the last page of this book. God's power knows no bound and it never goes on vacation. Always available for whoever believes. There is no particular day that God has programmed for your healing, as many wrongly think and continue to suffer. The day you believe is the God steps in and heals you. So call now if you believe, tell us whatever is harassing your and that devil will know there is a Living God in Heaven who has anointed vessels on earth to torment the tormentor. Just believe.

You can also call us to teach your people healing. Healing is one of the missing gifts and blessings of redemption missing in the church of Jesus Christ today. That is why Christians nowadays enjoy sickness more than unbelievers, which ought not to be so. We are always available to labor in our Father's vineyard both to bring in the lost and to bless the redeemed. In whichever way you need us, whether for a crusade, a seminar or healing conference in your church or city, feel free to call us now, and if God approves and sends us, we shall be there.

As you pray the prayers in part three of this book, do not bother where you are found. Just be sure you are in Christ and believe.

VII-   UNFORGIVENESS IS DANGEROUS

For if ye forgive men their trespasses, your heavenly Father will also forgive you: But if ye forgive not men their trespasses, neither will your Father forgive your trespasses, Matthew 6: 14-15.

Shouldest not thou also have HAD COMPASSION on thy FELLOWSERVANT, even AS I HAD PITY on thee?

So likewise shall my heavenly Father do also unto you, if ye FROM YOUR HEARTS FORGIVE not everyone his brother THEIR TRESPASSES. Mathieu 18: 33, 35.

PUT ON therefore, as the elect of God, holy and beloved, BOWELS OF MERCIES, KINDNESS, humbleness of mind, meekness, longsuffering; FORBEARING ONE ANOTHER, and FORGIVING ONE ANOTHER, if any man have a quarrel against any: even AS CHRIST FORGAVE YOU, SO ALSO DO YE. And ABOVE all these things put on CHARITY, which is the bond of perfectness, Colossians 3: 12-14.

God will not forgive those who refuse to forgive others, whatever their motives and reasons. Without forgiveness and the mercy of God, no one can and should expect answers to his prayers, it doesn't matter how much he suffers and cry in that situation.

Hatred, self-centeredness and pride are some of the things that prevent us most often from forgiving people. That is why we are recommended to put on **"BOWELS OF MERCIES, kindness, HUMILITY, gentleness and patience and charity"**,

That is to say, God's love, the love that gives, shares and forgives freely. So learn to forgive.

Unforgiveness is a sin, and it is one of the things that open door to some deadly afflictions.

Decide now to forgive those your rebellious and stubborn children who have abused you, your friends, your colleagues, your boss, your employees, your parents, and all those who have offended you, no matter their crimes and the gravity of their offenses against you. This is not an easy thing, but it is indispensable and commanded. It is not an option; God demands it and we all must do it.

Above all, forgive yourself first for your past. You need to forgive yourself of all your errors and mistakes that you have committed in life. For God said, **"Remember ye not the former things, neither consider the things of old. Behold, I will do a new thing; now it shall spring forth; shall ye not know it? I will**

even make a way in the wilderness, and rivers in the desert", Isaiah 43: 18-19.

Making a way in the wilderness here means, even if your life has no meaning or shape, if you have no one in life, if everybody has deserted and isolated you in your situation, God can and will change your story without any man's help. The wilderness talks of despair and hopelessness. He will give you hope and a solution where there is not even a grain of hope. Only believe, and forgive all those who have ruined your life. Be strong and courageous, your God is alive and He asking you: **"Can a woman forget her sucking child, that she should not have compassion on the son of her womb? yea, they may forget, YET WILL I NOT FORGET THEE. Behold, I have graven thee upon the palms of my hands..."** Isaiah 49: 15-16. A time came in David's life that everybody deserted him, but listen to what he tells us (Psalm 27: 10) **"When my father and my mother forsake me, then the LORD will take me up."** When I received Christ, I was rejected and despised. But by the revelation and encouragement of **Isaiah 49: 15**, I refused to give up my hope and faith. Today, my story has completely changed after about six years in the wilderness. God has now made me a light and a blessing to the nations. God will do the same for you as you look up to Him in faith in Jesus' Name. O there was a man called Joseph whom the brothers hated and sold him to slavery after beating him as their own appreciation for bringing them food. They beat him and threw him in the ditch, after filling their stomachs with the food he brought for them, they brought him out and sold him to the Ishmaelite and took him to Egypt, where he also was threw in jail for refusing to sin against his God. But when he had the chance to pay it back, he chose to forgive and show them love (**Genesis 42: 18, 50: 15-21).** Whatever a man does to you and on you can never equal nor alter God's plans and purposes in your life. A man may hate you and put dirty water on your white shirt, or even burn or tear your certificate, but will he also pour water on God's book and agenda concerning your life? Will he also tear or burn what God has written concerning you? Forgive whoever for whatever, and God will fight for you.

VIII- THE ATTITUDE OF PRAISE AND THANKSGIVING

Rejoice evermore. Pray without ceasing. In everything give thanks: for this is the will of God in Christ Jesus concerning you, 1 Thessalonians 5: 16-18.

Offer unto God thanksgiving; and pay thy vows unto the most High: And call upon me in the day of trouble: I will deliver thee, and thou shalt glorify me, Psalms 50: 14-15

THANKSGIVING is thanking the Lord for who He is, for what He has done and for everything we have received from Him.

Thanksgiving is an attitude, it is a spirit. It is the attitude of always recognizing God's works and blessings and thanking Him for them all. Avoid always looking at what you do not have or what others have. Comparison is a killer of gratitude, and ingratitude is a digger of grave. We must learn to consider and appreciate what we have that others don't have and may never possess because you are special and unique in the whole universe. Accept your personality, appreciate your uniqueness and always thank God for what you have, even just for the fact that you are alive.

If your feet or legs hurt, still thank God that you even have legs that hurt and you have a head to think. Many around you do not have the chance to walk every day like you on their two feet. Many have a head like you, but they feed in the trash bin because they are void of common sense and reasoning that God has freely given. Others have good heads, but cannot hear the good music and all the nice things you hear every day, or see the colors, the beautiful nature, football matches and movies that your eyes behold every day. Let's not always be ingrates grumblers, who complain, and are unhappy and unsatisfied no matter what God does for them and around them. When you keep complaining for what God has not done, never recognizing and appreciating what He has already done, you shut His ears from hearing your prayers, and bind His hands from saving you.

Impatience is one of the reasons why people don't thank God. I counseled a sister one day after the youth meeting who was so disgruntled. She was actually on fast since two weeks, but so full of complaints and bitterness that I advised her to stop the fast first. She complained about all her maids who are married, yet no man is asking about her. She complained about her musical album that has been on a still for more than a year, and complained about her family that is persecuting her, yet God is doing nothing about it. She complained about how she has been following and serving God for nine years, and how she has been living chastely yet God seemed to have forsaken her and closed hears to her cry. I took time to talk with her but she was so downcast that for hours we could not really get anywhere. At the end, I told her she lacked faith and trust in God. This sister was suffering of impatience, comparison, bitterness and faithlessness. So I just knew even her fasting, no matter the length could not move God to act. So I advised her to go and stop the fast, and praise God for one week morning and evening. Unfortunately the next day when I asked her, she told me she was not able to praise God, yet she is a singer. During the counseling session, I programmed a day of praise with her, but as I went home, my spirit was not free about it, so I cancelled it.

There are many like this sister who are so discouraged and hopeless that God is unable to do anything on their behalf. I reminded this sister of Sarah who had to wait for 25 years for the promised seed, and Joseph who was in the drain for almost thirteen years, yet he served and feared God without murmuring. Remember that without joy we can't draw any water out of the well of salvation **(Isaiah 12: 3)**. So be joyful and thankful to God. Sickness or any situation you find yourself does not mean that God has forsaken you and that you have sinned. What sin did Joseph commit? Yet he was sold into slavery and cast into jail upon that.

Was God not with him, even in prison? Read Genesis 39 very well. Did Jesus not love Mary and Martha? Did they commit any sin? Yet their only brother who Jesus also loved fell sick, and eventually died. They sent for the Master but he never showed up until after he has been four days in the tomb. When the Master with whom there is no impossibility appeared in the scene, He told them, **'Do not mourn, do not complain whether I came at your time or not, if only you can dare believe, then will you see the glory of the Lord though it seems all hope is lost'** (John 11: 40).

As they agreed with Him by their faith, He lifted up His eyes and engaged the mystery of thanksgiving: **"And Jesus lifted up his eyes, and said, Father, I thank thee that thou hast heard me," Vs 41**. Hell could no more contend Lazarus.

So your God is not dead, He is alive forever. Thank Him for the gift of life and for the good plans He has for you.

PRAISE on the other hand, is singing and praising God for who He is and what He has already done. It is also appreciating and singing hymns and songs to God for what He can do, what He has promised us as we recognize His power and goodness towards us.

Praise is an act of faith in our dead situation. Praising God in anticipation to what we want Him to do for us. It is actually celebrating the revelation of God's promises. That is why only men of revelation and understanding can truly praise God. For 25 years, Abraham was strong in the faith, giving glory to God for His promises to him and to his seed (Romans 4: 18-21).

"Is any among you afflicted? Let him pray. Is any merry? Let him sing psalms" Jacques 5: 13.

There is a time to pray and a time to sing psalms. Singing is for the merry-hearted. Until you develop and cultivate joy and contentment, you cannot sing.

Oh that men would praise the LORD for his goodness, and for his wonderful works to the children of men! For he hath broken the gates of brass, and cut the bars of iron in sunder...He sent his word, and healed them, and delivered them from their destructions. Oh that men would praise the LORD for his goodness, and for his wonderful works to the children of men! And let them sacrifice the sacrifices of thanksgiving, and declare his works with rejoicing, Psalms 107: 15-22.

Praise ye the LORD. Sing unto the LORD a new song, and his praise in the congregation of saints. Let Israel rejoice in him that made him: let the children of Zion be joyful in their King. Let them praise his name in the dance: let them sing praises unto him with the timbrel and harp. For the LORD taketh pleasure in his people: he will beautify the meek with salvation. Let the saints be joyful in glory: let them sing aloud upon their beds. Let the high praises of God be in their mouth, and a twoedged sword in their hand; Psalms 149: 1-9.

Learn to praise God. Many religious folks wonder why we sing and dance in the church and make some joyful noises. My dear, it is a godly noise of victory and triumph. This is to declare our victory over our enemies and circumstances. It is also inviting God into the scene, and when He comes He takes over and fights for us, defends us, and executes vengeance on our enemies as Psalm 149 says. Do you really want to know why this noise every time we gather in the sanctuary of our God? Because dead may be all around us, we may be tossed to and fro by the winds and storms of life, we may be pressed on every side, we may be opposed and accused, **"But thanks be to God, which giveth us the victory through our Lord Jesus Christ" – "Now thanks be unto God, which always causeth us to triumph in Christ, and maketh manifest the savour of his knowledge by us in every place" (1 Corinthians 15: 57; 2 Corinthians 2: 14).**

So with this understanding and assurance that your sickness is not unto death, you praise God. With the confidence and faith in the scriptures that I will at last come out victorious and triumphant however the case may appear in the eyes, I praise my Jehovah, the I AM that I AM; who inhabits the praises on His saints. God will never inhabit our tears and sorrows, He inhabits our praises. So give up that pitiable and miserable look, and smile. Praise Him earnestly.

When certain situations and problems confront you, engage yourself in high praises and God Himself will fight for you. Listen to this:

Then there came some that told Jehoshaphat, saying, There cometh a great multitude against thee from beyond the sea on this side Syria; and, behold, they be Hazazon-tamar, which is En-gedi. And Jehoshaphat feared, and set himself to seek the LORD, and proclaimed a fast throughout all Judah ... And when he had consulted with the people, he appointed singers unto the LORD, and that should praise the beauty of holiness, as they went out before the army, and to say, Praise the LORD; for his mercy endureth forever. And when they began to sing and to praise, the LORD set ambushments against the children of Ammon, Moab, and mount Seir, which were come against Judah; and they were smitten... And when Judah came toward the watch tower in the wilderness, they looked unto the multitude, and, behold, they were dead bodies fallen to the earth, and none escaped, 2 Chronicles 20: 2-3, 21-22, 24.

Faced with a company of three nations bigger and better armed (equipped) than him, Jehoshaphat cried out to His Great and Mighty God, **"O our God, wilt thou not judge them? for we have no might against this great company that cometh against us; neither know we what to do: but our eyes are upon thee"**(verse 12).

He did not just pray and folded his arm and watched. He prayed and praised. Inspired by the Spirit of God, he engaged the instrument of praise that never fails. Even if you're lying on the bed right now, sing some hymns to God from a sincere heart and if you can dance, go ahead: sing, clap for God, dance and jump in your situation by faith, and you will see the glory of God in your life, and His vengeance on your enemies.

PART THREE

RISE UP AND PRAY:

HOW TO PRAY FOR HEALING?

Luke 18: 1, 7-8: **And he spake a parable unto them to this end, that men ought always to pray, and not to faint... And shall not God avenge his own elect, which cry day and night unto him, though he bear long with them? I tell you that he will avenge them speedily. Nevertheless when the Son of man cometh, shall he find faith on the earth?**

Psalms 50: 14-15: **Offer unto God thanksgiving... And call upon me in the day of trouble: I will deliver thee, and thou shalt glorify me**

Psalms 91: 15-16: **He shall call upon me, and I will answer him: I will be with him in trouble; I will deliver him, and honour him. With long life will I satisfy him, and shew him my salvation.**

Mark 10: 27 **And Jesus looking upon them saith, With men it is impossible, but not with God: for with God all things are possible.**

Mark 11: 24 **Therefore I say unto you, What things soever ye desire, when ye pray, believe that ye receive them,**

and ye shall have them.

DO YOU BELIEVE?

Remember that it is not prayer that heals, but faith in the God to whom you pray. Before you pray, believe God will do it for you. And after praying, believe that God has done it.

Faith works in three stages, and in all three stages your faith is indispensable to obtain whatever you need:

BEFORE PRAYING

Before praying be sure and convicted that God will give you exactly what you ask, because He is faithful to His word. Remember the women with the issue of blood? She went to get healed and not see if she could be healed. Many pray hoping that God will do it if He chooses to. That is wrong attitude. Of course God is supreme, and might choose not to answer some of our prayers, depending on His will about the issue. But dear, about healing, we already know it is His will that I get healed and live healthy. In fact, you need without fail to read out books titled **DIVINE HEALING IS STILL POSSIBLE and WHY MUST I BECOME A CHRISTIAN Vol. 1 book 2.** At all cost locate these books or contact us for your copies, especially the one healing. Do not forgo these books for any reason.

Yes, God's will and sovereignty overrides our desires. However, it does not cancel our faith. Especially when it comes to divine healing, He wants us to live well and in peace. His mind about our healing and sound health is found all over the Holy Bible. But **Exodus 23: 25** and **3 John 2** are very clear about it.

So pray to be healed. Do not pray hoping that God will heal you as many do and miss their miracle. Rather, pray knowing and expecting God to heal you as you so desire like this woman: **And, behold, a woman, which was diseased with an issue of blood twelve years, came behind *him,* and touched the hem of his garment: For SHE SAID WITHIN herself, If I may but touch his garment, I SHALL BE WHOLE. But Jesus turned him about, and when he saw her, he said, Daughter, be of good comfort; THY FAITH HATH MADE THEE WHOLE. And the woman was made whole from that hour.** Mat 9: 20.

Before coming to the Master, this afflicted woman determined to be healed. She needed nothing but healing and total deliverance. For SHE **SAID** WITHIN herself, **"If I may but touch his garment, I SHALL BE WHOLE"**. And Jesus recommended her for her faith; confidence and assurance. By her faith she drew the virtue power from the master and got healed on the spot. You too can do the same.

WHILE PRAYING

As pray, maintain faith within you. Your inner man has a voice, which is very indispensable for your success and victory in any aspect of your life. As man thinks in his heart so is he. Be convicted and sure that God is hearing while you pray. Whether you feel anything or not, be sure that the devil is leaving your life.

The woman came **SAIYING WITHIN herself, If I may but touch his garment, I SHALL BE WHOLE.**

As you pray, the thought in your hearts are very important. Many say they believe, meanwhile within themselves they are wondering if they will at all be healed. They are praying and wondering at the same time on the inside if at all it will work for them. That is doubt.

The thoughts of our hearts have a lot to do with our prayers. Whatever you are praying for, not only healing, you need to believe what you saying, and say what you are believing God for. You need to mean what you are saying and say what you mean; what is on the inside.

Jesus told his disciples, "Have faith in God! I tell you with certainty, if anyone says to this mountain, 'Be lifted up and thrown into the sea,' IF HE DOESN'T DOUBT IN HIS HEART but believes that what he says will happen, it will be done for him. Mark 11: 22-23. (ISV)

Now if any of you lacks wisdom, he should ask God, WHO GIVES TO EVERYONE GENEROUSLY without a rebuke, and it will be given to him. BUT HE MUST ASK IN FAITH, without any doubts, for the one who has doubts is like a wave of the sea that is driven and tossed by the wind. Such a person should not expect to receive anything from the Lord. James 1: 5-17 (ISV)

During prayers, your faith must stay alive and strong. Your conviction on the inside must be fuelled up to burn up the beast of illness in your flesh.

He is in essence saying (in the above reference) that if the one praying doesn't doubt in His heart, he will have whatever he says. It is not about what you feel, but about what you believe. The word of your mouth must conform to the words of your heart. Remember God reads the heart and reads the thoughts of our hearts. Besides, that sickness inside of you, it senses also what is going on within you.

AFTER PRAYING

That is why I tell you, whatever you ask for in prayer, believe that you have received it and it will be yours. Mark 11: 24.

After you are done praying, do not wait to feel like healed. Believe you have received the requested healing. Ignore the symptoms. Jesus said; **You will receive whatever you ask for in prayer, if you believe.** Mat 21: 22 (ISV)
If you believe, you will get anything you ask for in prayer.

Mat 21: 22 (ERV)

And all things whatsoever ye shall ask in prayer, believing, ye shall receive. Mat 21: 22 (Darby)
As you follow these three stages of faith, adding to it what you have learned from this book so far, be sure you are free from Whatever you have suffering from. Today is your day of total freedom in Jesus Mighty Name. Amen!

Prayer 1

[Lord Jesus, thank you for dying for me on the cross. Come into my life and save me. Forgive me my sins, blot out my name from the book of death, and write it in your book of life and make me a child of God. I receive you this day as my only Lord and Savior in the Mighty name of Jesus Christ. Fill me with your Spirit now as promised to those who believe and who ask of it. I receive in now by faith in the Name of Jesus, Amen! Thank you Lord, for saving me from sin, from Satan and death to serve the Living God, for I am now a child of God.

Hear my prayer, O God, hear my supplication and grant me the desire of my heart. Deliver me now from doubt and unbelief, and answer me. O God of Glory, have mercy on me. You did not create me to suffer and be tormented by sicknesses and infirmities. Your Word says in Psalm 103 verse 3 that You forgive all my iniquities, all my sins and heal all my diseases, whatever their origin, their cause and their names. You are so good that you cannot deny me good things. Thank you Lord Jesus for taking all my infirmities and diseases. By your stripes I am healed. I accept and receive my healing that You paid the price more than 2000 years ago. I believe that by your death on the cross, all my sins are forgiven and I am made righteous and holy by Your blood through faith in You. I also believe and agree that by Your death on the cross Thou hast received the judgment and punishment that I deserve so that now I can have peace of mind, of the soul and body.

I also believe Lord and I accept that the stripes that led to your shameful death on the tree were for my total healing from all sicknesses and infirmities. So now I am healed of this disease (mention the name of the illness, and repeat this paragraph seven times). I declare and decree that I am healed in the Mighty Name of Jesus Christ of Nazareth. Amen!

You illness, you infirmity (mention the name), I order you: leave my body now and immediately, because Jesus took you and you're nailed to the cross. By His stripes I am healed in the Almighty Name of Jesus Christ. Amen! You unclean spirit afflicting me with (mention the name of the disease), I condemn you and curse you today in the Mighty Name of Jesus Christ. Perish and be uprooted now by fire and cleansed away by the blood of Jesus.

It is written in Isaiah 53: 4-5, "Surely he hath borne our [MY] griefs, and carried our [MY] sorrows: yet we did esteem him stricken, smitten of God, and afflicted. But he was wounded for our [MY] transgressions, he was bruised for our [MY] iniquities: the chastisement of our [MY] peace was upon him; and with his stripes we are [I AM] healed" So I declare all afflictions, pains and infirmities illegal/strangers in my life and my body. It is also written "And the inhabitant shall not say, I am sick: the people that dwell therein shall be forgiven their iniquity" (Isaiah 33: 24). **I will no longer be sick and I will never again say I'm sick, because my sins are forgiven and all my diseases are healed and removed in the Mighty Name of Jesus. Amen!]**

Now, open your Bible and read the following passages seven times a day for seven consecutive days. If you do not have a Bible (or if you have only the New Testament), buy a complete Bible now, even if it means to sell your TV or some of your clothes or shoes to buy one. The Bible is the first thing that every man on earth should have in his life, especially Christians. Have a Bible for yourself, buy one for your parents, your children and your wife. Keep one Bible in your office or shop and another at home. When travelling, the Bible should be the first thing in your bag, and make sure you read it constantly.

So, open your Bible and read the following passages seven times a day for seven consecutive days:
Psalms 103: 1-5, Isaiah 53: 4-6, Matthew 8: 16-17, 1 Peter 2: 24, Matthew 9: 35, Exodus 15: 26, Exodus 23: 25. If the person sick is unable to read, get his attention and read these passages to his hearing with confidence and authority.

Prayer 2

"And said, If thou wilt diligently hearken to the voice of the LORD thy God, and wilt do that which is right in his sight, and wilt give ear to his commandments, and keep all his statutes, I will put none of these diseases upon thee, which I have brought upon the Egyptians: for I AM the LORD that HEALETH THEE" Exodus 15: 26

"Bless the LORD, O my soul: and all that is within me, bless His holy name. Bless the LORD, O my soul, and forget not all His benefits: Who forgiveth all thine iniquities; who healeth all thy diseases" Psalms 103: 1-3.

Before praying, calmly consider the above passages, also read and confess **Mathew 8: 16-17** and **1 Peter 2: 24** seven times. **[O God, I praise You for You are good and faithful. Thou art the Lord that healeth me. I celebrate thy Holy Name and Your faithfulness because You are He who forgives all my sins and heals all my diseases without exception in the Name of Jesus Christ. O God of my salvation, merciful Father, hear me today, hear my prayers and grant me the desire of my heart in the name of Jesus Christ. I sincerely desire to live peacefully and in Health according to Your plans for me and my family in Jesus' Name. Deliver me now from doubt and unbelief and hear me now.**

O God of Glory, have mercy on me. You did not create me to suffer and be tortured by disease and infirmity. Your word says in Psalm 103 verse 3 that you forgive all my

transgressions, all my sins and heal all my diseases, whatever their source, their causes and their names. You are so good that you cannot deny me the good things of life. Your word says in Exodus 15 verse 26 that You are the God; the Lord who heals me. You do not lie and never change. Visit me my God and heal me now in Mighty Name of Jesus. Deliver me from this disease and affliction of the devil (mention the name of the disease). I declare my healing according to Thy word in the Mighty Name of Jesus.

O God, You are the Almighty Healer, in You I trust. Heal me and I will serve you. Deliver me from every sickness and infirmity and grant me good health in the name of Jesus. By the blood of Jesus Christ purge and, cleans my system and heal me completely. Send Your fire into my system, in my organism, and throughout all my body to burn every weed and chaff of sickness that the enemy has planted in my body in the Powerful Name of Jesus. I command, every infection, virus and bacteria in my system and in my blood, die now in the Mighty Name of Jesus. Amen! I receive my healing and my deliverance now in the Mighty Name of Jesus. Amen! Thank you Lord for hearing and healing me, because I believe I am whole now in Jesus' Name. Amen!]

Prayer 3

"**And the inhabitant shall not say, I am sick: the people that dwell therein shall be forgiven their iniquity**" (Isaiah 33: 24).

The people of Jerusalem here speak of Christian; the redeemed of the Lord. The church of Jesus Christ is Zion, the capital city of Jerusalem; the dwelling of Jehovah our Great God. That is where the temple of the Lord was located in the old time. But in another sense, Jerusalem is we ourselves; and our families, our home or where we dwell. For the temple of God was in Jerusalem, now we are His temple where His Spirit dwells.

In the New Testament when Jesus entered Jerusalem, He chased out the temple of God, all the sellers and money changers. We are that temple, if truly we have repented and received Christ as our Lord and Savior. Likewise, when He enters and settles within us, He chases every stranger in the name of sickness and disease.

We are the spiritual Jerusalem; the New Jerusalem coming out from God, a temple not made with hands. We are the dwelling place of the Living God. The Spirit of God now lives in us, no more in an arch or in a temple build of earthly materials as in the Old Testament. We who are born again are the living tabernacle of the Living and Clean God

Now concerning the Spiritually Jerusalem which we are, we are told in Revelation 21: **And I John saw the holy city, NEW**

JERUSALEM, coming down from God out of heaven, **PREPARED as a bride adorned for her husband. And I heard a great voice out of heaven saying, Behold, THE TABERNACLE OF GOD IS WITH men, and HE WILL DWELL WITH THEM, and THEY shall be HIS PEOPLE, and God himself shall be with them, and be their God. And God shall wipe away all tears from their eyes; and there shall be NO MORE DEATH, NEITHER SORROW, NOR CRYING, NEITHER SHALL THERE BE ANY MORE PAIN: for the former things are passed away"** (Verse 2-4).

This is true and certain, provided we believe it. Why "**NOR CRYING, NEITHER SHALL THERE BE ANY MORE PAIN"**? Because by the sacrificial death of Jesus Christ our Lord and Savior on the cross, **"Surely he hath borne our griefs, and carried our sorrows... he was wounded for our transgressions, he was bruised for our iniquities: the chastisement of our peace was upon him; and with his stripes we are healed. All we like sheep have gone astray; we have turned everyone to his own way; and the LORD hath laid on him the iniquity of us all"** (Isaiah 53: 4-6). So then, **"...if any man be in Christ, he is a new creature: old things are passed away; behold, all things are become new"** (2 Corinthians 5: 17).

Read again the following passages and receive your healing as you believe in Jesus Name:

Who hath believed our report? and to whom is the arm

of the LORD revealed?...Surely He hath borne our griefs, and carried our sorrows... He was wounded for our transgressions, He was bruised for our iniquities: the chastisement of our peace was upon Him; and with His stripes we are healed. All we like sheep have gone astray; we have turned everyone to his own way; and the LORD hath laid on Him the iniquity of us all (Isaiah 53: 4-6)

When the even was come, they brought unto Him many that were possessed with devils: and He cast out the spirits with His word, and healed all that were sick: That it might be fulfilled which was spoken by Esaias the prophet, saying, Himself took our infirmities, and bare our sicknesses, Mathew 8: 16-17.

[O God, you are the King of kings, the Almighty Savior of my soul and of my body. I thank you because my old things are passed away, including my sicknesses and sufferings, for it were my sorrows and my grief that Jesus took on His body, and it were my sicknesses and infirmities that He carried. I believe and I claim my total healing and deliverance in the Mighty Name of Jesus.

O God, by your Mighty hand, visit me and deliver me completely from the works of the devil. O Lord of Glory, heal me from all afflictions and sicknesses in my life now. Let every infection, bacteria and virus in my body and in my system die now in the Name of Jesus Christ.

O Lord, your word never lies nor fails, it is written by His stripes I am healed. So I believe it and I declare that by the stripes of Jesus I have been healed. By His blood I am purged, cleansed and set free. By His stripes I am completely healed.

I declare in the Name of Jesus, I am healed. I am healed and delivered from the power of satan and sicknesses on the Mighty Name of Jesus Christ. Amen. I am healed of this affliction (mention it) in the Name of Jesus. Amen!

You sickness, (mention it), I curse you and uproot you from my body in the Name of Jesus Christ. Be destroyed completely from my system in the Name of Jesus.

You unclean spirit of infirmity, I command you in the Name of Jesus Christ, leave my body. Jesus Christ my Savior overcame and defeated you on His cross, and in His Name every knee bows, therefore in the Name of Jesus, I command you, pack your luggage of sicknesses and depart from my body in Jesus Name. I am free from your power and bondage from now on in Jesus Name. Thank you Jesus for healing me. Glory to your Name forever more. Amen!]

Prayer 4

Thou shalt be blessed above all people: there shall not be male or female barren among you, or among your cattle. And the LORD will TAKE AWAY from THEE All SICKNESS, and will put none of the evil diseases of Egypt, which thou knowest, upon thee; but will lay them upon all them that hate thee, Deuteronomy 7: 14-15.

Beloved, I wish above all things that thou mayest prosper AND BE IN HEALTH, even as thy soul prospereth, 3 John 2.

For I know the thoughts that I think toward you, saith the LORD, THOUGHTS OF PEACE, and NOT OF EVIL, to GIVE you an EXPECTED END, Jeremiah 29: 11.

According to Deuteronomy chapter 7, verses 14 and 15, we are to be blessed and spared from sicknesses. Why? Because all His plans and thoughts for us are **"THOUGHTS OF PEACE, and NOT OF EVIL, to GIVE you an EXPECTED END"**. That is why His highest wish for you is "**that thou mayest prosper AND BE IN HEALTH, even as thy soul prospereth**". God has in project your happiness, your health and good success in life. Many believe that Christians are to suffer all their lives on earth and be happy only in Heaven. No. That is ignorance. If so be the case, why then did Christ suffer? In vain? No! No!

I agree and acknowledge that we must face challenges and difficulties down on earth, what do the scriptures have to say on this matter?

But thanks be to God, which giveth us the victory through our Lord Jesus Christ, 1 Corinthians 15: 57.

Now thanks be unto God, which always causeth us to triumph in Christ, and maketh manifest the savour of his knowledge by us in every place, 2 Corinthians 2: 14.

Should I still suffer the same things with unbelievers and sinners? I don't think so. Do you know that Christ came to bring many sons to glory? I am one of them. **"For it became him, for whom are all things, and by whom are all things, IN BRINGING MANY SONS UNTO GLORY, to make the captain of their salvation perfect through sufferings"**, Hebrews 2: 10.

So tell me, what glory is there in sickness, hunger and poverty? Why are many Africans and other people taking untold risks and sacrificing huge sums of money to run to Europe and America? Why don't they go to Ethiopia or Iraq? Is it not because every human aspire for a comfortable, peaceful and happy living? And that is the life Christ Jesus has to offer us here on earth. That is His offer for you and I here on earth and in Heaven above in the days to come.

Truly I feel sad for those who despise God's blessedness in

Christ and all those who belong to no church and enter no church in their life. Sorry for those who will not read their Bibles and discover God's wonderful promises to make living profitable and better for them on the earth. Without discovery of what said and did for you, there is no recovery of your inheritance in Christ. It is the discovery of what Christ accomplished for you on the cross that determines the recovery of your rights in Christ. Are you ready to lay hold of your inheritance of healing and good health in Christ? Then you must rise up with holy anger, and by faith against anything oppressing you and making life miserable for you. Whatever the issue, God can handle it as you pray and call it by name. Pray the following prayer with determination to get your freedom:

[Our Father who art on Heaven, the Great and Mighty God who lives in us by your Holy Ghost, be praised and glorified in the Name of Jesus Christ. You are holy and awesome in your works. I thank you for your unending and unconditional love for me. I thank you for your loving-kindness and mercy towards me and my family. Thank you Father because you desire above all things that I prosper and be in good health. Thank you O Great God for your plans of peace and comfort you have for me in Christ according to your word. Your word is sure and settled in Heaven forever and ever, and you never fail.

O Lord you are good and merciful. You are faithful.

Yes Lord of Glory, you are wonderfully good, Great and Mighty. And nothing has ever passed you when men believe in you. That is why I confidently put my trust and hope in you, for haling and comfortable living. And I know you cannot fail me in Jesus Name.

O God, visit my situation and avenge me from the power of (mention whatever be your trouble). You promised me in Deuteronomy 7:14-15, that you will bless me, heal me and put upon me none of the evil diseases around. I know sickness is evil and is not from you. Heal me Father in the Name of Jesus and restore my health.

Your word says in Mathew 15:13 that every plant you did not plant in my life shall be rooted out. Therefore I command every seed and plant of sickness in my life to be rooted out and burnt by fire in the Name of Jesus Christ.

(Now, place your right hand or your two hands on the concerned part as you continue)

You seed and plant of sickness, be completely rooted out of my life now in the Name of Jesus. You seed and planting of sickness and afflictions in my family, be completely rooted out now in the Mighty Name of Jesus Christ. You seed and planting of cancer, fever, diabetes, Aids, of bareness, high blood pressure, hypertension, of tuberculosis...be burnt now by fire in the Name of Jesus, and never you return again for it is written, 'whosoever the son of man shall set free is free indeed. I declare that I am free from your power and I will live and testify the goodness of my God unto old age.

Thank you dear Lord, for healing and completely delivering me from the yoke of this sickness and diseases in the Name of Jesus. I love you and I promise to follow and serve you the rest of my life in health, in peace, in joy, happiness and prosperity by the Holy Ghost in the Name of Jesus Christ. Amen!]

Prayer 5

Who Himself bore our sins in his own body on the tree, that we, having dead to sins, might live for righteousness- by WHOSE STRIPES you WERE HEALED, 1 Peter 2: 24
Stand fast therefore in the LIBERTY wherewith CHRIST HATH MADE US FREE, and be not entangled again with the yoke of bondage, Galatians 5: 1
If the SON therefore shall MAKE YOU FREE, ye shall be FREE INDEED, John 8: 36.

The Son of God did not die in vain. He died for a reason: to free us from the yoke of sin and its wages which are sicknesses and death. Sin makes man a slave of Satan, but when Christ enters into our world, He destroys everything that is from satan, beginning with diseases. **"He who sins is of the devil; for the devil has sinned from the beginning. For this purpose the Son of God was manifested, that he might destroy the works of the devil"**, 1 John 3:8. We understand from Acts 10:38 that the devil oppresses people with diseases but Jesus delivers and heals them by the anointing of the Holy Spirit: **"how God Anointed Jesus of Nazareth with the Holy Spirit and with power, who went about DOING GOOD HEALING ALL who were oppressed by the devil, for God was with Him."** So, pray and be released from the power of the devil in Jesus' Name. Amen! Sickness is an oppression of the devil.

[Lord Jesus, I thank You for paying the price for my liberty and making me free indeed through faith in Thy cross. Thank you because I know you still go about doing good well and healing all those who have faith in you, for God is in your as He was with you about two thousand years. So take Your place in my life and heal me now in Jesus' Name.

Holy Spirit divine, who quickens and gives life to our mortal and dying bodies, I acknowledge that You are glorious and good. I thank You because You have a mission from God to make life comfortable and peaceful for me. You're the comforter and helper of the saints in the light. Take Your place in my life Holy Spirit Divine and quicken me in the name of Jesus Christ. Deliver me completely from everything that makes my life miserable, bitter and uncomfortable in the Name

of Jesus Christ. Deliver my life from the pit and torment of satan. Holy Spirit, I open my heart to You, I offer You my body as a living sacrifice, holy and pleasing to God, I am Your temple. Install yourself and sweep Your house. By your fan, clean completely my system and my body from all that offend. According to Matthew chapter 3 verse 12, Thou hast Thy fan in thy hand to sweeps and clean Your floor (your temple) and to burn up the chaff with unquenchable fire, the fire that burns and consumes everything on its path as the fire of Elijah. My body is your holy temple, and by your fan and by your fire, cleans and purify my body from all filthiness of disability and burn completely every chaff of sickness and disease in the Mighty Name of Jesus. Amen!

Heavenly Father, thank you for the fire of your Spirit, whose mission is my glorification. By the anointing of Your Spirit, break every yoke of disease and infirmity in my life in Jesus Name. By Your Fire, accomplish Your projects/plans of peace, of total healing and divine health in my life in the Mighty Name of Jesus Christ. Thank you father for you have heard and answered me. I believe and accept that I am saved and healed in Jesus' Name. Amen!]

Accept your healing now by faith and begin to appreciate God the Father, the Son and the Holy Spirit for their perfect work in your life. It is done in the Name of Jesus. Amen!

Prayer 6

Ask, and it shall be given you; seek, and ye shall find; knock, and it shall be opened unto you. For EVERY ONE THAT ASKETH RECEIVETH; and he that seeketh findeth; and to him that knocketh it shall be opened ... If ye then, being evil, know how to give good gifts unto your children, how much more shall YOUR FATHER which is in heaven GIVE GOOD THINGS to THEM THAT ASK HIM?, Matthew 7: 7-8, 11.

And whatsoever ye shall ASK IN MY NAME, that will I do, that the Father may be glorified in the Son. If ye shall ASK ANY THING in MY NAME, I will do it, John 14: 13-14.

Healing and health is good but God gives good things only to those of His children who ask Him. Let us remember that Jesus went from place to place doing good, according to **Acts chapter 10 verse 38**. Healing is that good He goes on doing, but we must ask in prayers by faith in His name.

Until now you have asked nothing in My Name. ASK and you shall receive, that your joy may be full, John 16: 24.

[O God, I come to You in the Name of Your Son Jesus Christ. Thank you for my salvation and my deliverance which Thou hast prepared in Christ from the foundation of the world

and that You executed by His death on the cross at Golgotha, and which are revealed to me in Your word. Lord, Your Name is a strong tower where I find refuge, safety and protection according to Proverbs 18:10 and Psalms 91:1. That is why I ask and I request for my healing and my total health package in that Name which is above any other name.

Lord Jesus, at the mentioning of Your Name every knee shall bow and every tongue confesses that You are Lord to the glory of the Father. You also say that whatever we ask in your name we will be given us. Therefore, by the authority and efficiency of your infallible word, I decree that my recovery is established in the Name of Jesus.

O God, deliver me from this malaise, deliver me from all afflictions and sicknesses and infirmities in the Name of Almighty Jesus. In the Name of Jesus Christ, I take my full recovery now.

You illness or disability, you unclean spirit of infirmity, be banished from my life in the Mighty Name of Jesus, stop oppressing my soul and tormenting my spirit by your burdens of disease and get away from me in the Name of Jesus Christ. Stop right now afflicting and weakening my body in the Powerful Name of Jesus. Release my health and my wealth which are mine in Christ, you devourer of good things in my life. In the Mighty Name of Jesus I condemn you and I bind you, get out and never come back. Go to the desert and perish, from this moment, I am no longer your slave, nor your

candidate, in the Name of Jesus Christ of Nazareth. Amen!
Amen! I am totally free. The Son of God has set me free, I am
free indeed, and I refuse to be still under the yoke of the enemy
in the Name of Jesus. O God of glory, thank you for your
goodness, thank you for healing me. Thank you Heavenly
Father, thank you for my release from the power and
oppression of Satan in the Name of Jesus Christ. Amen!]

Prayer 7 - against sicknesses with wounds or injuries, and tumors.

Therefore all they that devour thee shall be devoured;
and all thine adversaries, every one of them, shall go into
captivity; and they that spoil thee shall be a spoil, and all that
prey upon thee will I give for a prey. For I will restore health
unto thee, and I will heal thee of thy wounds, saith the LORD;
because they called thee an Outcast, saying, This is Zion, whom
no man seeketh after, Jeremiah 30: 16-17.

Praise ye the LORD: for it is good to sing praises unto our
God; for it is pleasant; and praise is comely. The LORD doth
build up Jerusalem: he gathereth together the outcasts of
Israel. He healeth the broken in heart, and BINDETH UP
THEIR WOUNDS, Psalms 147: 1-3.

Behold, happy is the man whom God correcteth: therefore
despise not thou the chastening of the Almighty: For he

75

maketh sore, and **BINDETH UP: HE WOUNDETH, and HIS HANDS MAKE WHOLE. He shall deliver thee in six troubles: yea, in seven there shall no evil touch thee,** Job 5: 17-19.

God also heals wounds and injuries; by the way some wounds are not natural. There are some wounds and injuries you cannot explain their sources and causes; that is why they defy any medication. Yet Jehovah has the final say. And Jesus is the Great physician and the Doctor of all doctors. Call Him by faith, and He will do what He alone can do. Before praying, you can apply some anointing oil around the wound or injury. If it is a tumor or pain, anoint the spot with oil and pray:

[O God, You who bind and heal our wound, I thank you because you're not a partial God. What You do for one you can do it for ten. What are you doing in Nigeria and Canada; you can also do it in Cameroon and China, that's why I magnify Thee with all my heart with confidence that you will do it for me too. O God, the Great Healer, You opened the eyes of the blind and raised the dead without number, and you have not changed. Jesus is the same yesterday, today and forever. Lord, heal my wounds. Heal my physical, mental, spiritual, emotional and psychological Wounds in the Mighty Name of Jesus Christ. O God, my eyes are on You for my total healing and complete and quick recovery in the Powerful Name of Jesus Christ. Your Word says that You bind my wounds and heal me by your hand. Therefore manifest Thy power and Thy strong hand to get me healed because Jesus Christ bore my

suffering and my pain, He was wounded for me and bruised for my iniquities that I might be healed and made whole in Him. I agree and declare that by His stripes I am healed completely in Jesus' Name.

(Impose now your right hand on the pain or wound and say): **You wound, you pain, you tumor ... enough is enough. In the Name of Jesus Christ, I command you to dry and disappear from my body. Jesus was wounded and bruised for me, now I curse in the Name of Jesus anything that holds you and keeps you on my body. I destroy thy power and thy roots in this body in the Powerful Name of Jesus Christ. Amen! Thank you Lord because I'm cured now. I believe you've already healed me and this wound, tumor and pain will dry away from my body in Jesus' Name. Amen!]**

Prayer 10: For servants of God (those serving God).

Every born again Christian must understand that he is God's servant. Therefore you have the right to the repair and servicing of your body and your whole system by the Holy Spirit who cleanses us by His fire and by the word of God that we receive in Zion (the Church of God). When you go to church and worship God, and help the Saints when you evangelize and sing for God, pray for the church, for souls, for your pastors, other believers, the nation, when you give your tithes and your offerings , and you help or assist your pastors, it is your and service contribution to the kingdom of God. And God has promised healing and health for His children. In addition, the Scriptures say that we cannot serve two masters at the same time. So, I cannot, and you must not serve God and sicknesses at the same time. I refused it, as you must also refuse it, because it's what we bind or refuse on earth that God refuses in Heaven **(Matthew 18: 18).** Do not accept or settle down with sickness and poverty. If you accept, God also approves. My body carries the Holy Spirit of God, and the unclean spirit of infirmity and disease has no place in me. It is the same for you. Do you know that every servant is entitled to a recompense or reward? **"And ye shall serve the LORD your God, and he shall bless thy bread, and thy water; and I will take sickness away from the midst of thee. There shall nothing cast their young, nor be barren, in thy land: the number of thy days I will fulfill "**, Exodus 23: 25. This passage literally means is that God will bless us with enough bread (good food in abundance) and water. **"Then shall ye return, and DISCERN between the righteous and the wicked, BETWEEN HIM THAT SERVETH GOD and him that serveth him not"**, Malachi 3: 18.

So, I must in no case suffer the same things and suffer the same diseases as sinners and non-Christians do. It is illegal. Before praying, read Luke 1: 68-75 seven times, 2 Corinthians 5: 1 and Romans 8: 1.

[My God and my King, I thank You for the privilege to

serve you. I glorify You because You are a rewarder of those who diligently seek You, and You are not unrighteous to forget the services of Thy servants. You are a just God who does no unrighteousness. O God, as I am in Your service, avenge me in Jesus' Name. Your word says that I will not serve two masters at the same time, so how can I serve You and sickness at the same time? O God, it is unfair and against Your nature and Your covenant. Visit my health and heal me in Jesus Name. Take away from me this evil infirmity, deliver my body of this disease in the Mighty Name of Jesus. You promised that I will be different from those that do not serve you, I do not have to suffer the same things as others; then my case is different. I am the apple of your eyes, and I am part of your body O Jesus of Nazareth. Lord, do as You promised me in Exodus 23 verse 25 to take away from me all sickness and all the works of Satan in Jesus' Name.

You disease and infirmity, get away from me with immediate effect in the Powerful Name of Jesus. You do not have the right to operate in this body. I curse and reject you now in the Mighty Name of Jesus Christ. Amen! By the stripes of Jesus, I am Healed. By the blood of Jesus I am saved and freed from your power satan, in the Mighty Name of Jesus. I am healed- I am healed -I am healed- I am healed-I am free, I am free, I am completely healed and free in the Name of Jesus Christ. Amen! Thank you Lord for having accomplished your promise, I receive my healing now in the Name of Jesus Christ. Thank you Lord, Thank You Lord, Thank you Jesus, Thank you Lord. Amen!]

John 5: 14 **Afterward Jesus findeth him in the temple, and said unto him, Behold, thou art made whole: sin no more, lest a worse thing come unto thee.**

Galatians 5: 1 **Stand fast therefore in the liberty wherewith Christ hath made us free, and be not entangled again with the yoke of bondage.**

PART FOUR

TOTAL DELIVRANCE:

FREEDOM FROM SPIRITS HUSBANDS (SEX IN DREAM), FOOD IN DREAM AND ALL FORM OF OPPRESSIONS.

But thanks be to God, which giveth us the victory through our Lord Jesus Christ, 1 Corinthians 15: 57.

Now thanks be unto God, which always causeth us to triumph in Christ, and maketh manifest the savour of his knowledge by us in every place, 2 Corinthians 2: 14.

Christ sets us free from all oppressions. As a Christian, understand that you are married to Christ. As the matter of fact, sex in dream is illegal. You dine with the Lord daily at His table, and food in dream is no permitted. The prayers in this section will help all those facing oppression and whatever sorts of afflictions in their Christian adventure. If you are not a born again child of God, please, be born again. Repent now and give your life to Christ. Pause now, and say the prayer of salvation at close of this section. If you are not a Christian, you can still get a miracle by calling on the Name of Jesus because every devil bows to that Name, but it will not take you to anywhere. It might do more harm than good as the devil will be back with his allies to torment you worse than ever before.

PRAYER ONE

[O God, I come to You in the Name of Your Son Jesus Christ. Thank you for my salvation and my deliverance which Thou hast prepared in Christ from the foundation of the world and that You executed by His death on the cross at Golgotha, and which are revealed to me in Your word. Lord, Your Name is a strong tower where I find refuge, safety and protection according to Proverbs 18:10 and Psalms 91:1. I command by your authority, let every power tormenting me to bow now and leave me now in Jesus Precious Name. It is over with this situation (mention it) I have been going through. That is why I ask and I request for my healing and my total health package in that Name which is above any other name.

Lord Jesus, at the mentioning of Your Name every knee shall bow and every tongue confesses that You are Lord to the glory of the Father. You also say that whatever we ask in your name we will be given us. Therefore, by the authority and efficiency of your infallible word, I decree that my recovery is established in the Name of Jesus. Amen!]

PRAYER TWO

[O God, deliver me from this malaise; deliver me from all afflictions and oppressions in the Powerful Name of Jesus. In the Name of Jesus Christ, I demand and I claim my full recovery now.

You spirit husband, you unclean spirit of infirmity, be banished from my life in the Mighty Name of Jesus, stop oppressing my soul and polluting my body and get away from me in the Name of Jesus Christ. I bind you now and stop your activities in my life in Jesus Name. Release my health and my wealth which are mine in Christ, you devourer of good things in my life. In the Mighty Name of Jesus I condemn you and I bind you, get out and never come back. Go to the desert and perish, from this moment, I am no more your wife. I can no longer dine with you. I am no longer your slave, nor your candidate, in the Name of Jesus Christ of Nazareth. Amen! Amen! I am totally free. The Son of God has set me free, I am free indeed, and I refuse to be still under the yoke of the enemy in the Name of Jesus. O God of glory, thank you for your goodness, thank you for healing me. Thank you Heavenly Father, thank you for my release from the power and oppression of Satan in the Name of Jesus Christ. Amen!]

PRAYER THREE

Lord God, I belong to you alone, or Your word says in Romans 7: 3-4, "A married woman, for example, is bound by the law to her husband as long as he lives; but if he dies, then she is free from the law that bound her to him. So then, if she lives with another man while her husband is alive, she will be called an adulteress; but if her husband dies, she is legally a free woman and does not commit adultery if she marries another man. That is how it is with you, my friends. As far as the Law is concerned, you also have died because you are part of the body of Christ; and now you belong to him who was raised from death in order that we might be useful in the service of God. "

Therefore, it is abnormal, and even illegal for me to eat in the dream, have sex in the dream with whomever. I refuse it and I declare an end to it today because am married to you, in the Name Jesus. I condemn every spirit husband (or wife) and spiritual husband (or wife) in my life, and I divorce myself from him spirit, soul and body in the Name of Jesus. I declare the divorce and I renounce all involvement and agreement between me and him (her) by the Name of Jesus. I invoke the light of God against every personality and every spirit that feeds me, or who sleeps with me at night. Holy Spirit of God, act in my life and wrap me with your fire day and night in the Name of Jesus Christ. Let all my oppressors be scattered by fire in Jesus' Name.

PRAYER FOUR

I am born of God. Lord Jesus, I thank you for having died for me on the cross to make me a child of God. O God, I praise you and I crown you the King of my life. Jesus is my Savior and my Redeemer. I am born of God; therefore I am out of reach of the devil and his agents. For it is written that whoever is born of God is preserved and the wicked one cannot touch him anymore, according to 1 John 5: 18. I believe in that, and I declare, I will no longer suffer from nightmares, food in the dream, night poison, sex in the dram, and all kinds of night attacks in the Name of Jesus. O God, let fire scatter and burn up everything bothering my life at night.

By the blood of Jesus, I destroy and disarm every weapon formed against me and my family, and all arrow prepared against me in dreams in the Name of Jesus Christ.

Let the fire of the Holy Spirit burn and neutralize everything they have deposited in my spirit, soul and body through the food and sex in the dream in the Name of Jesus. I have the life of God in me, I have eternal life. It is over with every act of wickedness on my life in Jesus' Name. Lord thank you, for giving me victory in every aspect of my life through the blood and the Name of Jesus Christ. Amen!

PRAYER AND CONFESSION

I declare: I believe in Jesus Christ, who died for me on the cross to take away my sins and bear my sorrow and my grief, He rose from the dead the third day to give me total victory over the enemy. I acknowledge that He suffered for me and His body was broken and wounded for me.

I acknowledge that He Himself bore MY sicknesses, and carried MY pains. He was wounded for my sins, and broken for my sins. The punishment that brings me free peace was upon Him, and by His stripes I am healed in Jesus' Name. Amen!

It is written, "Give thanks to the Father, who has made us meet to be partakers of the inheritance of the saints in light, who has delivered us from the power of darkness and conveyed us into the kingdom of His dear Son: in whom we have redemption, the forgiveness of sins." (Colossians 1: 12-14). I believe and I declare that I am delivered from the power of Satan and his demons.

Satan, demons and witches have no more power over me. I cannot suffer sexual harassments in dream again; I am out of reach of spiritual (and spirit) husbands as from now on, and I will no more eat in dream. Satan and witches can no more torment me and oppress me day or night, for he who is born of God does not sin, he keeps himself and the wicked one cannot touch, according to 1 John 5: 18. No evil has power over me any longer. I am preserved. In Jesus Christ all my sins are forgiven me and deleted because according to Isaiah 53: 5, "He was wounded for my sins, bruised for my iniquities", and in Colossians 1: 14, in Him I have "redemption and the forgiveness of all my sins." I believe in Jesus and I am saved. Old things are passed away, now everything is become new in my life.

PRAYER FIVE: AGAINST DEMONIC OPPREESSIONS OR SICKNESSES

Giving thanks unto the Father, which hath made us meet to be partakers of the inheritance of the saints in light, which WE ISSUED A power of darkness and brought us into the kingdom TRANSPORTED of his beloved Son, in whom WE REDEMPTION, the forgiveness of sins, Colossians 1: 12-14. He who sins is of the devil, for the devil has sinned from the beginning. The Son of God appeared was to DESTROY THE WORKS OF THE DEVIL, 1 John 3: 8.

There are some diseases and afflictions that we cannot explain. They come and go, often at specific times of the year or month.

For some, it is when they receive their salary or an important sum of money, or when they undertake a project or an important event in their lives that a certain misfortune or illness attack them and devour everything. It is as if the disease had ears and eyes. For some women, it is when they are in their ovulation period that mysterious things happen. Some get pregnant, and a man sleeps with then in dream and the nest thing they see is blood. When that happens, the pregnancy vanishes away.

These are in most cases mystical diseases caused by witches and evil men (not far from us). Or a demonic disease, that is, caused by a demon. In both cases, a demon or evil spirit has been assigned in the life of that person to reduce his life to nothing and ruin his finances, in order to induce him or her to misery and misfortune throughout his life. But the word of God tells us that JESUS CHRIST **"the Son of God came for this: TO DESTROY THE DEVIL'S WORK "** (1 John 3: 8).

Through our faith in Christ and our new birth into His Kingdom, God delivers us from the power of the devil and his agents, and takes us into the New Jerusalem, which is the Kingdom of His dear Son. So whatever the affliction in your life disease and its source, you have to be set free. In my childhood, I suffered of different manners of diseases that no one could tell the name, and no witchdoctor or sacrifice was able to deliver me. I cannot count how many traditional doctors I was taken to, in my country and in remote villages, and the sacrifices made to so-called ancestors. Nothing went well until Christ came into my life. Praise Jehovah RAPHAH!

Christ has me completely free and delivered and healed. Today, I am truly free. You too can live sickness-free. God did not create you with that disease that has become your life partner. God did not create you to live on a diet due to illness. God did not create you with hypertension or diabetes. Even if all your ancestors have had it, even if everyone in your family or lineage suffers from a particular disease or affliction, you can be different if you just cross over into Jesus' camp. Make up your mind to divorce the disease, tell it goodbye. Today is your salvation in the Name of Jesus Christ. I declare you free and blessed. Amen! Go ahead and pray:

[Heavenly Father, You are Almighty God, and no one can fight with you. Nobody has ever resisted your right hand. Pharaoh tried it and was reduced to nothing with his whole army. Goliath tried it and was brought down Holy! Holy! Holy is Your Name. Wonderful and terrible are thy works, O God Almighty. You act according to Your good will and nobody can resist your powerful hand acting on behalf of the saints on earth. O God be praised, be exalted, be magnified in Your holiness. You are a God of justice and who in revenge pour your wrath on your enemies. LORD of hosts, I invoke Thee this day, I stand before the throne of grace through the Name of Your Son Jesus Christ, our Lord and my Redeemer. Vindicate me, O God of Glory and I will declare thy wonderful works among the people, I will tell Your goodness and faithfulness to the saints. Lord God, there is nothing too hard for you and nothing is above you. O God, a day came and you changed the story of Anne, grant me this day my total deliverance in Jesus Name. Enough is enough for this situation in my life (mention the issue as you pray). This is too much. I'm tired and fed up with the sorrows of this life, and you promised in Matthew 11 verse 28 to give rest to those who come to You. Do it for me, O Jehovah Raphah! O Jehovah Nissi, you are faithful and powerful.

O my God and my Father, The righteous cry, and the LORD hears, and delivers them out of all their troubles! Deliver me from whatever resists Your glory and Your wonders in my life. By your fire, act in my life and deliver me

from the power and control of any stubborn demon in the Mighty Name of Jesus. At the mention of the Name of Jesus every knee must bow. I command every knee to bow in my life, in Jesus' Name. I order all stubborn and resistant afflictions in my life to fleex and disappear in the Name of the Lord Jesus Christ.

You sorrow and affliction, I order you now, disappear from my life now in the Name of Jesus, loose your power over my life in Jesus' Name. Be completely destroyed in the Name of Jesus Christ. I refuse to die in this affliction. I break the power of death and the grave of my life in the Powerful Name of Jesus. I cancel any order and any plan of premature death about my life and my family in the Name of Jesus Christ of Nazareth. I return to the sender any bad news prepared for me and my family in the Powerful Name of Jesus. Like king David; my ancestor in the faith, I declare that I will live well and die "in a good old age, full of days, riches, and honor" in the Mighty Name of Jesus. I pull my life and health out of the hands of my captors now in Jesus' Name.

O Holy Spirit of God, take possession and total control of my life and put my enemies to flight in permanently in the Name of Jesus Christ. Amen! Thank you Lord, for thou hast heard me, and hast set me free. I am loosed and totally free in the Name of Jesus. Amen!]

PRAYER DURING PREGNANCY

(ESPECIALLY FOR DIFFICULT OR UNSTABLE PREGNANCIES)$

Place your hands on your belly before praying and repeat over and over until delivery. Often anoint your stomach with anointing oil before praying. If you have already decided the name of your child, which I advise you to do, call his/her name from time to time, and bless him.

[Children are a reward from the Lord, children are a blessing, and the blessing of God makes rich and happy, He adds no sorrow to it, according to Proverbs 10: 22. So I declare that my pregnancy is a blessing, my baby is a source of joy and happiness, and not of sorrow and pains. I will give birth to my baby without problems, even before labor comes. I will deliver my child through normal process. The God who gave me this child is with me, and His Mighty Hand is upon me always will until delivery. It is written, "Before Zion was in labor, she gave birth; before she was in pain, she delivered a boy. Who has heard of such a thing? Who has seen such things? Can a land be born in one day or a nation be delivered in an instant? Yet as soon as Zion was in labor, she gave birth to her sons. "Will I bring a baby to the point of birth and not deliver [it]?" says the LORD; "or will I who deliver, close [the womb]?" says your God. Be glad for Jerusalem and rejoice over her, all who love her. Rejoice greatly with her, all who mourn over her", according to Isaiah 66:7-10 (HCSB). I am the woman the Bible is talking about. I declare that any weapon formed against me and my baby will have no effect, it shall not prosper. I decree by the Holy Spirit, "Before I travailed, before I am in labor, I have brought forth my child." I declare and decree with insurance in the Powerful Name of Jesus Christ, before my pain came, I have given birth to my child. The word of God does not lie, God is committed to fulfill His word in my life. So I declare in the Precious Name of Jesus Christ, as soon as I am in labor, I, the daughter of Zion, give birth to my healthy son! The Lord is my shepherd, I will fear nothing. He is with me, so

everything will be fine. Thank you Lord Jesus, for Your powerful Hand on my life now and forever. I surrender myself to you, because I know you cannot disappoint me.
O God, arise and act in my life. I give myself entirely to you this day, and I choose to follow you the rest of my life, and abandon the life of sin. Lord Jesus, hear me and come to my rescue. Today I have chosen you as my master and my husband. Sanctify and cleanse me with Your precious Blood, deliver me from the power of Satan, demons and sin to serve the living God. I receive the Holy Spirit into my life, to walk in the truth and worship in spirit and in truth you.]

NOW STAND FIRM

FINALLY, MY BRETHREN, BE STRONG IN THE LORD, and in the power of his might. Put on the whole armour of God, that ye may be able to stand against the wiles of the devil. For we wrestle not against flesh and blood, but against principalities, against powers, against the rulers of the darkness of this world, against spiritual wickedness in high places. Wherefore take unto you the whole armour of God, THAT YE MAY BE ABLE TO WITHSTAND IN THE EVIL DAY, AND HAVING DONE ALL, TO STAND. STAND THEREFORE, having your loins girt about with truth, and having on the breastplate of righteousness; And your feet shod with the preparation of the gospel of peace; Above all, taking the shield of faith, wherewith ye shall be able to quench all the fiery darts of the wicked. And take the helmet of salvation, and the sword of the Spirit, which is the word of God: Praying always with all prayer and supplication in the Spirit, and watching thereunto with all perseverance and supplication for all saints, Ephesians 6: 10-18.

Learn to resist sickness and all afflictions of the devil. Nothing settles in your without your permission. The problem is neither with God, nor the devil. You are the problem. If you make your mind to live healthy, you can. To ride on over the devil and live a victorious and triumphant Christian life, you must locate a living and Spirit-filled church, and abide there. Do not follow religion, do not follow the church because someone has brought you there or because it is a family church, but because you are convicted God is there. Be there because you are taught God's word. I am not saying you should not follow your family to the same church, but be careful not to follow people in error and you know it. Seek God personally and have a relationship with Him out of love and sincerity.

Also, get your copy of our books **"DIVINE HEALING IS STILL POSSIBLE"**, and **"WHO IS A CHRISTIAN"**, by the same author, and you will greatly be blessed. Feel free also to contact us for help and counseling.

But most importantly, understand that God is not responsible of your mediocre living, and it is not holiness. Satan is your problem, if does anything in your life it is because you allow Him. Look at what happened in the garden of Eden. When man fell, God knew very well how it happened. But he asked man, because satan was not supposed to operate. It was man's duty to put the devil where he belongs, and control the garden as God had charged him.

Your health, your marriage, your business, your finances, education, children, etc, are what constitute your garden, and it is your responsibility to determine what happens to it. I am talking to those in Christ.

In the garden, **"And the LORD God planted a garden**

eastward in Eden; and there he put the man whom he had formed... And the LORD God took the man, and put him into the garden of Eden to DRESS it and to KEEP it" Genesis 2: 8; 15

To dress means to put it in order and in good shape. To KEEP it means to control and watch over. It was not satan that was given charge over the garden, but man. Now, look at what happened (Matthew 13: 24-28, 38-37);

Another parable put he forth unto them, saying, The kingdom of heaven is likened unto a man which sowed GOOD SEED in his field: But WHILE MEN SLEPT, his enemy came and sowed tares among the wheat, and went his way. But when the blade was sprung up, and brought forth fruit, then appeared the tares also. So the servants of the householder came and said unto him, Sir, didst not thou sow good seed in thy field? from whence then hath it tares? He said unto them, An enemy hath done this...He answered and said unto them, HE THAT SOWETH THE GOOD SEED IS THE SON OF MAN ...The enemy that sowed them is the DEVIL".

If you sleep over your life, and health, be ready for tares. Now, when Christ came, He gave unto us what it takes to dominate and have the last say over our health, and entire life on earth;

Luke 10: 19 **Behold, I give unto you power to tread on serpents and scorpions, and over all the power of the enemy:**

and nothing shall by any means hurt you.

That is why you are called to resist him; that is, to stop him from sowing tares in your life. Jesus will not come and resist him for you. Neither Mary, nor his angels will come and tread over his power for you, you have to.

RESIST HIM

Behold, I give unto you power to tread on serpents and scorpions, and over all the power of the enemy: and nothing shall by any means hurt you. Luke 10: 19

Be sober, be vigilant; because your adversary the devil, as a roaring lion, walketh about, seeking whom he may devour: Whom resist stedfast in the faith, knowing that the same afflictions are accomplished in your brethren that are in the world, 1 Peter 5: 8-9.

Jesus did not say He will come and tread upon serpents and scorpions for you, neither did He say He will send His angels to win over all the power of the enemy for you. He said you are the one to do it by the power He has given unto you, as you become a born again Christian. So rise up and use the power given unto you to ride over sicknesses and diseases. You know, many Christians think that satan is so powerful that he can afflict them at will and make them ill, not so for me. You have been raised over him. You are the son of GOD. You have power and authority over and his demons and agents.

He has no more pore, nor authority. He has been spoilt and disarmed:

And Jesus came and spake unto them, saying, ALL

power is given unto me in heaven and in earth. Matthew 28: 18

Colossians 2: 13-15 **And you, being dead in your sins and the uncircumcision of your flesh, hath he quickened together with him, having forgiven you all trespasses; Blotting out the handwriting of ordinances that was against us, which was contrary to us, and took it out of the way, nailing it to his cross; And having spoiled principalities and powers, he made a shew of them openly, triumphing over them in it.**

We believe this book has being a real blessing to you. We also pray that this book becomes a powerful tool in your hands in setting the captives free wherever you may be found. May you graduate from healing to sound health. By this book, May the Lord of hosts convert you into a healer and terror for satan and sickness. You are highly favored. We will be glad as you call us or write for your testimonies and even for prayer and counseling. Feel free. Above all, introduce this book to as many as you can, and the Lord will bless you great. It will be great also if you invest a few dollars to buy copies for your loved ones and for some sick people around you. Visit the hospital and the prison and buy them some copies and guess what? God will in no way forget your gesture:

God is fair, and he will remember all the work you have done. He will remember that you showed your love to him by helping his people and that you continue to help them. We want each of you to be willing and eager to show your love like that the rest of your life. Then you will be sure to get what you hope for; Hebrews 6: 10-11. **God is not unfair. He will not forget the work you did or the love**

you showed for him in the help you gave and are still giving to other Christians, Our great desire is that each of you keep up your eagerness to the end, so that the things you hope for will come true; Hebrews 6: 10-11.

Then the King will say to the people on his right, 'Come, you that are blessed by my Father! Come and possess the kingdom which has been prepared for you ever since the creation of the world. I was hungry and you fed me, thirsty and you gave me a drink; I was a stranger and you received me in your homes, naked and you clothed me; I was sick and you took care of me, in prison and you visited me.' The righteous will then answer him, 'When, Lord, did we ever see you hungry and feed you, or thirsty and give you a drink? When did we ever see you a stranger and welcome you in our homes, or naked and clothe you? When did we ever see you sick or in prison, and visit you?' The King will reply, 'I tell you, whenever you did this for one of the least important of these followers of mine, you did it for me!' Mat 25: 34-40

LETTER TO THE READER

Dear reader, we love you. We would love to meet you in Heaven. How wonderful will it be when we all meet in His banquet hall as the bribe of the Son of the Living God to celebrate as the angels and all the heavenly hosts gaze and rejoice for final victory!

Strive to live healthy and to overcome the devil and his agents, but above all forgo everything else to make Heaven. We recommend you our other book titled **"DIVINE HEALING IS STILL POSSIBLE"**, which is the continuation of this one. It is rich, loaded, insightful and impactful. This one is just the introduction to it.

Some of our books include: **MORNING SHOWER** (a daily devotional), **DIVINE HEALING IS STILL POSSIBLE...** Vol. 1, **WHO IS a CHRISTIAN-WHY MUST I BE a CHRISTIAN** –Vol. 1 (book 1 & 2), Vol. 2, **THE GOOD SHEPHERD, THE EFFECTIVE PRAYER OF THE BELIEVER, DANGEROUS PRAYERS.**

You need to read these books. Are you a minister of the Gospel, a Christian worker, a new convert, a churchgoer or an unbeliever, you need them. Many are in the church for years, but all they can tell you is that Christianity is to escape from hell. Many have failed to embrace the God of Christianity because they wonder why they should change their beliefs. In these books, the Holy Spirit exposes to the reader some clear reasons why you must become a Christian. It will help also help all Christian workers passionate for soul winning. They will constitute powerful tools in your hands for effective evangelism. Other books in view include **THE EFFECTIVE PRAYER OF THE BELIEVER, DANGEROUS PRAYERS**, and many more.

Stay blessed and strong in the grace of the Lord!

I love you dearly;

PRINCE HUBERT TATANG

ABOUT THE AUTHOR

PRINCE HUBERT TATANG; is an ordained minister of Jesus Christ, a young missionary called by God and trained in China. He began fulltime missionary service in 2007, and has ever since been instrumental in the hands of God in the mission field in Africa, precisely in Cameroon and Nigeria.

Prince Hubert is a Tele and Radio evangelist, and teacher in seminar and conference Speaker. He is a teacher on marriage and healing.

His is a writer and author of several books including **MORNING SHOWER** (a daily devotional), **DIVINE HEALING IS STILL POSSIBLE..."** Volume 1 & 2, **"WHO IS a CHRISTIAN-WHY MUST I BECOME a CHRISTIAN"** (Volume 1 book 1 & 2, and Volume 2), **THE GOOD SHEPHERD, WINNING THE WAR AGAINST SICKNESS,** and many others.

Contact the Author:

+237- 79 71 62 90
+237- 94 07 51 32.
princeofj@gmail.com

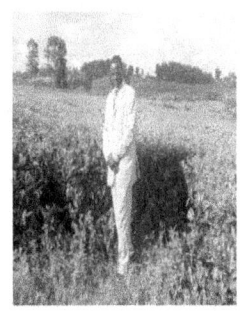

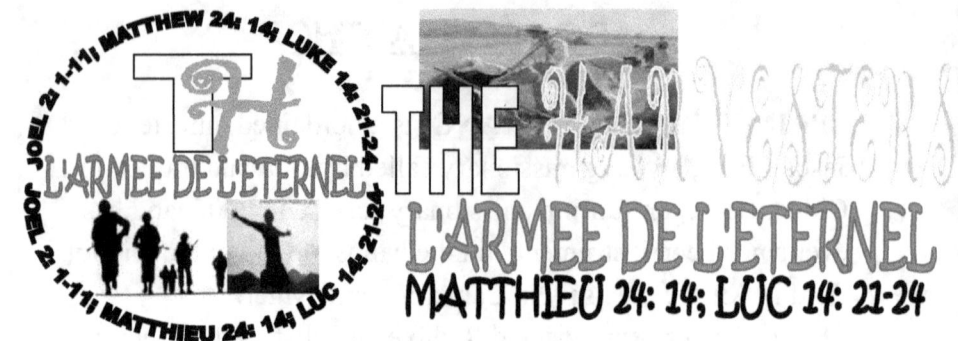

THE HARVERSTERS A.K.A. THE ARMY OF THE LORD
Joel 2:1-11; Matthew 24: 14; Luke 14: 21-24

Our Mission: Spread the Gospel, fill the earth with the knowledge of the Lord (Is 11: 9), snatching souls from hell into the Kingdom of lights

Our Vision: Take the light of the Gospel into villagers, to remote and unreached areas, get into schools and universities, get into hospitals and reap men out of hell by the preaching of the Gospel.

Strategy: Use the Media (TV, Radio, internet…), crusades, literature/tracts, CDs, seminars, medical outreaches…

"The Harvesters", also known as **"The Army of The Lord"** is an army of the redeemed of the Lord from every field of life, from any church across the globe who are willing to live for Him who died for them, **" that they which live should not henceforth live unto themselves, but unto him which died for them, and**

rose again", 2 Corinthians 5: 15.

This is the great end-time army who have laid down their lives, time, talents and resources for the vast and speedy spread of the Gospel, gathering multitudes into His banquet hall before His great return,**"a great people and a strong; there hath not been ever the like, neither shall be any more after it, even to the years of many generations... as a strong people set in battle array. Before their face the people shall be much pained: all faces shall gather blackness. They shall run like mighty men...they shall not break their ranks: Neither shall one thrust another; they shall walk everyone in his path: and when they fall upon the sword, they shall not be wounded. They shall run to and fro in the city; they shall run upon the wall... The earth shall quake before them... And the LORD shall utter his voice before his army: for his camp is very great: for he is strong that executeth his word"**

Many have heard the Gospel, many are yet to hear and be saved, and be harvested into His house before His return, **"So that servant came, and shewed his lord these things. Then the master of the house being angry said to his servant, Go out quickly into the streets and lanes of the city, and bring in hither the poor, and the maimed, and the halt, and the blind. And the servant said, Lord, it is done as thou hast commanded, and yet there is room. And the lord said unto the servant, Go out into the highways and hedges, and compel them to come in, that my house may be filled".**

As David rightly said, **"the work is great because the temple is not for man"**- **1 Chronicles 29: 1.**

This vision is only for those who believe that all those who die around them and far away have no hope in eternity, thus are ready and eager to cross their church walls and snatch a soul from hell.

Do you want to see souls saved? Are called to missions? Are you moved to give your time and resources to win a soul? Then this vision is for you whatever your location and distance...

You can work or partner with this vision in various ways.

Feel free to contact us or even call in others to join **"THE HARVESTERS".**

Tel: +237-79 71 62 90; +237-94 07 51 32 - princeof@gmail.com

www.ingramcontent.com/pod-product-compliance
Lightning Source LLC
Chambersburg PA
CBHW070932290526
45795CB00001B/493